FIRESIDE

Also by Doris J. Rapp

**Questions and Answers about Allergies
and Your Child**

Allergies and the Hyperactive Child

by Doris J. Rapp, M.D.

A FIRESIDE BOOK
Published by Simon & Schuster Inc.
New York London Toronto Sydney Tokyo Singapore

Manufactured in the United States of America

7 8 9 10

Library of Congress Cataloging in Publication Data

ISBN: 0-671-61131-3

To my mother
whose ever positive attitude
encouraged me to study medicine

Acknowledgments

I wish to thank the following physicians, Albert Rowe, Theron Randolph, Frederick Speer and William Deamer, for their recognition of multiple adverse body responses to foods. I regret that I did not believe what you had written many years ago. Theron Randolph deserves special praise for his pioneering observations of the deleterious effects of chemical contamination and pollution. His writings were at least forty years ahead of the times. I wish to thank Joseph Miller, as well as Tenno Mae Lunceford, Francis Waickman, and John and Tina MacLennan for the awakening, the sharing and the helping, as I struggled to learn the practical applications of clinical ecology. My total skepticism was not easily subdued.

I would also like to thank Mary Ann Klepp and Sharon Steele for secretarial help and Lucy Wargo for helping with library research.

Contents

Foreword

As a pediatric allergist, I have seen many allergic children who were hyperactive and who were, in many cases, behavior problems. Often, improvement in their activity seemed to parallel improvement in their allergic problems. Fortunately for these children, the main problem was allergy which responded to standard allergy management after an allergist was consulted.

What about those children whose primary problem is hyperactivity? Is their problem also allergic? Whom should parents consult for diagnosis? What treatment is available? Should parents put their children on an elimination diet, and for how long? What should parents expect from such a program?

The possible role of food allergies and other intolerances in hyperactivity has recently been given much publicity. Research has been sometimes difficult to evaluate and medical opinions have differed. The mechanism of action in this relationship remains unknown. *Allergies and the Hyperactive Child* is the most complete book I know of on this subject and it gives parents, for the first time, a means to evaluate the controversy for themselves.

Dr. Rapp offers parents a practical treatment alternative, one that eliminates possible causes rather than treating symptoms with medication. Obviously not all hyperactivity is food or allergy related. Symptoms may not respond to dietary adjustment; even so, parents of hyperactive children will appreciate this added information as an aid to deciding what course of action to take for the greatest chance of success. In order to decide wisely you must be informed. As a physician, I believe this is the greatest contribution of *Allergies and the Hyperactive Child*. I am sure I will want to refer to it frequently.

James P. Kemp, M.D.
Associate Clinical Professor of Pediatrics
University of California–San Diego

Preface

When we think about allergy, we usually conjure up an image of sneezing, runny noses; itchy, tearing eyes; wheezing and coughing; or rashes. Less commonly recognized symptoms include muscle aches, headaches, dizziness, fatigue.

What about children, and adults, who are often depressed or irritable, overly active, belligerent, or poor learners? You may know, or may be the parent of, a child who is hard to discipline, continually disruptive, and barely accepted by peers and siblings because of hostile and erratic behavior. Some allergists and pediatricians believe these symptoms also can be due to allergies.

As a pediatric allergist, I began to notice that some children treated for allergies appeared to have fewer behavior and activity problems. Patients treated for hayfever, asthma, or eczema improved dramatically in disposition. Their activity levels sometimes seemed more normal and their schoolwork improved. Some parents also noted that their children's chronic muscle aches, legaches and headaches subsided.

Early in 1976, I decided to attempt a special study of a group of children previously diagnosed as being hyperactive. These preliminary studies appear to show a relationship between food sensitivities and hyperactivity. Ongoing studies indicate that diet can modify hyperactivity and behavior in *some* children who appear to have food allergy. Further long range, well designed scientific studies are obviously essential to evaluate and explain this apparent relationship.

In the meanwhile, this nontechnical book was written to help educate parents of hyperactive and/or allergic children about this possible relationship. It answers the obvious questions about these two medical problems and presents a simple one-week diet that can be used by parents to determine if food treatment will alleviate the behavioral or learning problems of their child. Such treatment may prove a welcome alternative to drug therapy and possibly reduce the expensive care needed from highly trained specialists.

Try the diet for one week and at the end of that time compare your child's activity and behavior before and after the diet. Has the condition improved? If so, you can proceed to determine the offending food items.

This book was written to help you, your child, and your family. Before following the suggestions, however, I recommend that you consult your physician. Your doctor knows your child's health problems and she or he alone can advise what is best.

Some patients may want to try this diet even though their doctor may disapprove. If the diet has not helped within fourteen days, do not continue it. In that case the diet suggested in this book is probably *not* the answer for your child. If the diet does help, however, be sure to discuss it with your physician. Prolonged diets without medical supervision can cause nutritional problems in children and adults.

Some physicians will be upset because this book was written before my medical research has been confirmed. I understand their skepticism and appreciate and respect the need for physicians to want solid medical and scientific support. Our priorities, however, must be in order. The one-week diet will not hurt anyone, and in my experience it appears to help a large number of children and adults quickly. To convince research-oriented physicians that the diet is effective will require years of rigorous testing. Because this subject presently generates so much controversy and negative feeling among some allergists, it may be difficult to obtain acceptable, valid, impartial research. It seems unreasonable and illogical to ask hyperactive children and their parents to wait ten years until we are sure. Children with activity, behavior, and learning problems should not suffer in the interim, especially when the treatment recommended will not be harmful and the answers may be two short weeks away.

Allergies
and the
Hyperactive Child

1 · The Relation of Allergy to Hyperactivity

This chapter briefly reviews medical reports, from 1908 to the present time, which indicate that a relationship between allergy and hyperactivity might exist. It discusses, briefly, some recent studies by others and myself concerning foods and hyperactivity.

Many parents, teachers, and physicians have asked: "Can something a child eats be related to activity, behavior, or learning problems?" The answer is, we simply don't know. There are some pediatricians and allergists who say: "Yes, I diagnose it all the time and help such children." There are other reputable physicians who authoritatively state that diet does not help. Do the ones who claim success actually help their patients? Have the ones who say children can't be helped by such means actually tried diets? Have they merely theorized and said diets can't help? Let's briefly review what's been said and done and try to come to sensible conclusions which might help parents and children in need.

THE MEDICAL LITERATURE

As early as 1908, reports were published in the medical literature stating that some children were noted to be fretful, irritable, restless, and unable to sleep if they ate certain foods (Schofield 1908, Schloss 1912, Cooke 1922, Hoobler 1916, Campbell 1927, Keston et al. 1935, Alvarez 1946, Black 1942). It was wondered if some children did not have an allergy that affected their brain or nervous system rather than the lungs (asthma) or nose (hay fever). Early investigators often described some patients as being extremely tired or fatigued rather than overactive; sometimes the same child was too tired at certain times and too hyperactive at other times (Randolph 1947, Rowe 1950, 1959). Others noted that foods seemed to change some children's behavior so that they acted depressed, hostile, or irritable (Alvarez 1946, Davison 1949, 1952). As the years passed, it was observed that pollens, dust, molds, and certain odors such as perfumes, could cause similar reactions in some patients (Speer 1954, Crook et al. 1961, Dickey 1971a, 1976a, b, Feingold 1975, Breneman 1978).

In 1930, Albert Rowe described a condition which he called "food toxemia." In a large book titled *Food Allergy*, he and his son recounted numerous patients who had drowsiness, irritability, fatigue, weakness, slowness, and inability to behave. He devised very strict diets which appeared to help many patients who had typical forms of allergy, as well as nervous-system problems, and he claimed almost unbelievable success. Some physicians attempting to duplicate his methods succeeded, others failed. Dr. Rowe firmly believed that foods, as well as pollens and dust, could contribute to psychological and nervous-system problems in some patients. He stressed the diets must be done correctly or patients might not improve, even though foods caused their medical problems.

During the 1940s and 1950s, more and more reports described similar patients. Dr. Theron Randolph, another author of many books and medical articles, described "allergic fatigue" (1947). He stressed that at times affected children and adults acted normal, but after eating certain foods or being exposed to offending odors or chemical substances, their behavior became distinctly abnormal. Some became very tired, others hyperactive. He noted affected individuals often had a rather pale face but were not anemic, and had swelling and black circles under their eyes.

THE ALLERGIC-TENSION-FATIGUE SYNDROME

In 1954, this term was coined by a prominent pediatric allergist, Dr. Frederic Speer of Kansas City. He recognized patients with symptoms similar to those described by physicians fifty years earlier. He edited a book for physicians on central-nervous-system allergy (1970). Dr. Speer and Dr. William Deamer of San Francisco, in many articles over the past thirty years, have repeatedly tried to make the medical profession more aware of this common problem. Through the years, the following symptoms have described patients affected with allergic-tension-fatigue syndrome.

ALLERGIC-TENSION-FATIGUE SYNDROME
Possibly includes any of the following

Nervous System Symptoms	Other Medical Symptoms
Hyperactive, wild, unrestrained	Nose: year-round stuffiness, watery
Talkative (explosive, stuttering,	nose, sneezing, nose-rubbing
constant)	Aches: head, back, neck, muscles, or
Inattentive, disruptive, impulsive	joints—i.e., "growing pains,"or
Short attention span	aches unrelated to exercise
Restless legs, finger tapping	Belly problems: bellyaches, nausea,
Clumsiness, incoordination, tremor	upset stomach, bloating, bad
Insomnia, nightmares, inability to	breath, gassy stomach, belching,
fall asleep	vomiting, diarrhea, constipation
Nervous, irritable, upset, short-	Bladder problems: wetting pants in
tempered	daytime or in bed, need to rush to
High strung, excitable, agitated	urinate, burning or pain with
Moody, tired, weak, weary, ex-	urination
hausted, listless, depressed	Face: pale, dark eye circles, puffiness
Easily moved to tears, easily hurt	below eyes
Highly sensitive to odor, light,	Glands: swelling of lymph nodes of
sound, pain, and cold	neck
	Ear problems: repeated formation of
	fluid behind eardrums, ringing
	ears, dizziness
	Excessive perspiration
	Low-grade fever

Some children are fatigued, tired, weak, mentally confused, irritable, drowsy, depressed, have body aches, fever, chills, and night sweats. These children often sleep poorly, awaken at night, have nightmares, and cry out in their sleep. Often they have learning problems.

Many children have associated nasal symptoms—a runny, watery nose, sneezing-in-bouts, nose rubbing, and wiggling. They have dark circles and puffiness or "bags" below their eyes, which can vary in intensity from day to day.

Many have constipation or diarrhea, vague bellyaches, appetite problems, and bad breath. (Milk and eggs, in particular, may cause the latter.)

While some children are fatigued and tired, others are overactive, restless, clumsy, and stutter. They are oversensitive to light, sound, pain, and discipline. They often cry. Some are cruel or may bully, fight, and hurt people. They have few friends.

These symptoms may not be constant. They not only vary from week to week and day to day, but sometimes from hour to hour. The cause is often related to a child's diet, so he may be adorable, then suddenly become impossible within a few minutes after eating.

Dr. William Crook's findings

In the early 1960s, Dr. William G. Crook of Tennessee, a pediatrician, attempted to make more pediatricians aware of this problem. He published an article in which he described fifty patients who appeared to have the allergic-tension-fatigue syndrome (1961). All but one had fatigue, irritability, mental or emotional symptoms, a pale face, circles under the eyes, and a congested nose. In addition, some of the group also complained of headache, stomachache, leg, back, or joint pain, excessive perspiration, low-grade fever, eye problems, bladder problems (day or night wetting or pain with urination), swelling of the abdomen, numb hands, tingling feelings, swollen hands, rapid or irregular heartbeats, and puffiness, swelling or soreness of the lips. He found that almost 75 percent of these children also had typical allergic symptoms, such as nose, chest or skin allergies (hay fever, asthma, eczema, or hives). He found that about 65 percent of the patients had relatives with typical allergies. He found that allergy skin-testing for foods, as it is traditionally done, did not always prove helpful in detecting foods that caused symptoms, but newer methods of food testing appeared to be reliable (see chapter 4).

Although foods were the major cause of symptoms in most patients he helped, some also appeared to be bothered by grass or ragweed pollen, dust, and horse hair or dandruff. The major foods causing the allergic-tension-fatigue syndrome in his patients appeared to be milk, chocolate, and eggs, although some were also sensitive to wheat, corn, peanut, pork, orange juice, and sugar.

In 1961, Dr. Crook performed one of the first double-blind studies to try to verify his findings. His patient is typical of those with this type of medical problem and, therefore, will be discussed in some detail.*

*From "Systemic Manifestations Due to Allergy," by W. G. Crook, W. E. Harrison, S. E. Crawford, and B. S. Emerson, in *Pediatrics*, vol. 27, page 794. © 1961 by the American Academy of Pediatrics, used with permission.

M. L. was born in 1944. He had an itchy skin rash called eczema when he was less than one year old and his parents noticed that the rash disappeared when milk was taken from his diet. For the next eight or nine years he had little difficulty except for nose stuffiness in the winter. He had occasional belly problems and periods when he seemed unusually fatigued and listless. In 1955, he first began to complain of headaches and frequent abdominal pain. He became cross, nervous, and irritable. His face was pale, he had dark circles under his eyes, and his lips appeared parched and swollen. He often had back and leg aches and seemed tired when he got out of bed in the morning. The diagnosis was a psychosomatic disturbance. At some point, his mother wondered if allergies could be a factor. Cow's milk and dust were found to cause positive allergy-skin-test reactions. He was placed on a milk-free diet and within a week he seemed to awaken refreshed and not tired, his stomachache and headache were gone, and his disposition improved. In the subsequent three years, whenever he drank milk or ate dairy products for several meals, he again became irritable, nervous, depressed, and had stomachaches and headaches.

To prove scientifically that this was truly a milk problem, Dr. Crook asked the child to swallow sixteen capsules a day for a period of thirty days. The patient did not know that during the first two weeks he was swallowing capsules that contained sugar, while for the second two weeks the capsules contained milk. Neither did Dr. Crook know which capsules were milk and which were sugar. This type of research is called a double-blind study because the physician, patient, and his family do not know exactly which food is hidden in which capsules. (When the physician, but not the patient, knows which of the coded capsules contains milk, it is called a single-blind study.) The patient kept daily records of how he felt, as did his parents. The child seemed normal till about the seventeenth day (after he had had milk-filled capsules for about three days) when fatigue and irritability reappeared; during the next week these problems worsened. He again developed stomachaches and headaches. Within forty-eight hours of stopping the milk-containing capsules, the youngster felt fine.

Dr. Crook subsequently wrote several books for the public to help them understand this problem more fully (1973, 1977, 1978).

Drs. Kittler and Baldwin's findings

In 1970, Kittler and Baldwin noted the similarity of symptoms in patients diagnosed as having minimal brain dysfunction (MBD) and those having the allergic-tension-fatigue syndrome. Twenty MBD children with abnormal electroencephalograms and a high incidence of allergy randomly were placed either on a diet composed of allergy-skin-test-positive or -negative foods. Impartial psychological evaluations showed an increase in intelligence scores in some children of normal intelligence during the diet which avoided skin-test-positive foods. Subjective teacher evaluations of behavior and objective readings of electroencephalograms also revealed improvement in some of the patients who avoided inhalants and probable food offenders. Evaluations were made without any knowledge of which patients were treated for allergies. The authors concluded that a significant percent of children diagnosed as MBD had allergy as the cause of their problem.

Dr. Ben Feingold's findings

The next major step in relation to hyperactivity was made by Dr. Ben F. Feingold of San Francisco. In 1975, he wrote a book entitled *Why Your Child Is Hyperactive*, which was publicized quickly throughout the nation. In this book, he states that he believes hyperactivity is mainly due to artificial food coloring, artificial flavors, and natural salicylates. Although he admits some children are also affected by other food items, dust, pets, pollens, and odors, he does not believe that allergy is directly related to hyperactivity. He describes how he became interested in this problem, the scope of hyperactivity and learning problems in this country, and includes a diet which he claims helps relieve symptoms in about 50 percent of affected children in one to three weeks. He says some children who eat dyed foods, for example, may have symptoms within two to four hours which can last for one to three days. As do Drs. Rowe (1950, 1959), Randolph (1947), Speer (1954), Crook (et al. 1961), and Deamer (and Frick 1972), he claims to have helped innumerable children using his special diet as a form of therapy.

Dr. Feingold is not only to be admired for making the public and physicians aware of this problem, but he and Dr. Stephen Lockey of Lancaster, Pennsylvania, have been particularly responsible for recent federal legislation so that the exact contents of foods in the United States will be labeled more specifically. This in turn has led to less contamination of processed foods with food additives, such as artificial colors and preservatives. Dr. Lockey has been a crusader pioneering against the dangers of artificially colored foods, beverages, and drugs since 1947.

The medical profession's response to observations concerning hyperactivity

At this point the medical profession, in general, is not pleased. Although well-meaning, honest physicians-in-practice claim hyperactive patients lose their symptoms on diets and have a recurrence of their problems when they stop the diet, this does not mean that there is a cause-and-effect relationship and certainly does not mean a patient has allergy. For example, you can develop diarrhea and bowel problems every time you drink milk and seem well when you don't, but this may not be a milk allergy. It could be due to a lack of a certain enzyme, such as lactase, in your intestines. So caution must be used in interpretation; this, however, does not alter the basic premise. It does appear that some unacceptable activity and behavior problems noted in some children are related to eating certain foods. To understand the role of foods scientifically, however, more double-blind studies are necessary. The medical profession rightly cautioned the public and physicians that more research and study of this problem is indicated. At present, at least two large federally funded studies are being conducted which "suggest" that a few patients might become hyperactive from food coloring (Wender 1977).

The value of a double-blind study

A double-blind study is designed to help eliminate prejudices on the part of both the patient and investigator. The experiment is designed so that the patient is given two items: one that is the real thing and another that looks and tastes like the real thing, but is not. This latter is called a placebo. The investigator has the two look-alikes coded by an impartial person, so only the coder knows which is which. The patient is then asked to try both coded items and tell the investigator which one helps. If the patient selects the real one, and not the placebo, it tends to indicate that the effect of the test item is probably real and not psychological or due to some unrelated factor.

Double-blind studies in relation to hyperactivity

Two psychologists, Drs. Keith Conners (et al. 1976) and J. Preston Harley (1976), each did a similar investigation in which they carefully studied hyperactive patients for a baseline period of one month before the children were placed on special diets. The children had several types of psychological and other tests to determine how they were "normally." They were then randomly and alternately placed on either a Feingold-like diet for one month or on another diet "which seemed equally difficult." After each diet, psychological tests and evaluations were repeated. In Dr. Conners' study both parents and teachers agreed that the Feingold-like diet reduced the children's activity compared to the baseline period. The teachers noted a few children who had highly significant reduction of symptoms during the Feingold-like diet, but not on the control diet. The parents, however, could not differentiate between the control and Feingold-like diet. The final results were, unfortunately, inconclusive, and subsequent research studies had to be designed.

An interesting point is that the few hyperactive children who improved were generally the ones who received the Feingold-like diet after the placebo diet. It is possible that when the Feingold-like diet was given first, the beneficial effect extended into the placebo diet period, obscuring proper evaluation of the diets, but that when the placebo diet was given first, the true effect of each diet was more obvious. Dr. A. Rowe (and Rowe 1972) and Dr. H. Rinkel (et al. 1951) pointed out years ago in their writings that if a patient were sensitive to a food and stopped eating it for three or more weeks, it was not unusual for the patient to remain well, even though he resumed eating the food again. After a few days or weeks, however, the sensitivity often recurred and the suspect food again caused symptoms. This observation helps to explain some of the confusion in the minds of many concerning why specific foods appear to cause symptoms on some occasions, but not on others. This problem is discussed further in regard to the history of Stephen below.

Subsequent studies by Drs. Charles Goyette and C. Keith Conners (Conners et al. 1976) have demonstrated that some parents can differentiate chocolate cookies which contain food coloring from those which do not, *if* they observe and rate their child's activity during the three-hour period *immediately after* the cookies are eaten. The cookies were prepared in a double-blind manner.

Other hyperactivity studies

In 1976, Dr. C. Hawley and Dr. R. Buckley from California studied one hundred patients and found that 40 percent reacted positively when tested with sublingual (under the tongue) food coloring. They found their patients responded favorably to a diet that restricted their intake of artificial food colors and salicylates. Two Australian investigators in 1976 published articles related to the Feingold Diet. Dr. P. Cook and Dr. J. Woodhill found that 66 percent of fifteen children responded favorably to the diet, and relapsed promptly when the diet was discontinued. Dr. L. Salzman studied thirty-one hyperactive children and found that 58 percent reacted positively when tested with sublingual food dyes. When fifteen of the dye-test-positive children were placed on the Feingold Diet, he found that 93 percent showed significant improvement within four weeks.

In 1977, Dr. Joseph Miller of Mobile, Alabama, reported a double-blind study of eight adults and children who had diverse symptoms. One four-year-old boy had marked hyperactivity, was restless, and had crying spells, a short attention span, and insomnia. Discipline was a problem at home and at school. He had an allergic face (see chapter 3). He wet his pants during the day and at night. He was skin-tested by an improved method (see chapter 4) for foods and received food-extract treatment in a double-blind manner for a period of eighty days. His symptoms persisted during the two twenty-day periods when he received the placebo therapy and subsided during the two alternate twenty-day periods when he received his food extract. Not only did his activity and behavior improve, but his sleep problems and urinary symptoms subsided.

In 1978, three English physicians recognized foods as a cause of behavior or nervous-system problems. Dr. Buisseret (1978) studied seventy-nine milk-allergic children with multiple complaints. Their symptoms repeatedly subsided when milk was omitted from their diets and recurred when it was ingested. He described twenty-seven patients as excessively nervous, timid, "high strung," aggressive, withdrawn, and prone to nightmares. Malingering was wrongly suspected in some children because their symptoms often occurred just before school. All children responded well to a milk free or individualized diet. Only 33 percent of the children had a positive allergy-skin-test reaction to milk but 84 percent reacted to other common allergenic substances. Allergy was noted in 86 percent of the families.

Drs. Finn and Cohen (1978) describe six patients who were chronically ill and not helped by any conventional form of medical care. Several patients were nervous, depressed, lethargic, and unable to work or study. In three patients a tube was passed from the patient's nose to the stomach. They were tube-fed different food items. On five occasions, in each patient, the offending item caused the problem symptoms, while placebo challenges with water or nonoffending food items caused no symptoms. Avoidance of the problem food items relieved diverse symptoms noted in all patients.

In 1978, Dr. I. J. Williams, and his associates in Ontario, Canada, studied the effects of randomly assigned active or placebo medications in combination with dye-containing versus placebo cookies. Double-blind evaluations by parents and teachers of twenty-six hyperactive children revealed that activity-modifying medications were more effective than diet. Approximately 25 percent of the children, however, did show reduced activity levels during the Feingold diet.

Dr. J. Preston Harley and others from the University of Wisconsin also reported on additives in 1978. A very elaborate detailed double-blind study of thirty-six school-age children failed to support any relationship between additives and hyperactivity. The study reported that while parents' behavioral ratings of ten hyperactive preschool boys indicated a favorable response to the diet which excluded artificial food colors, flavors, salicylates and some additives, laboratory observation and neuropsychological data could not confirm the parents' impression of improvement. All patients were placed on two diets. These were given in a double-blind manner over a period of six to eight weeks. To ensure compliance, *all* foods were supplied for families, visiting relatives or friends and home or school parties during the entire study.

In both studies it was assumed that the amount of artificial color in one of the two diets contained an amount of food coloring equal to the average daily diet of children in the United States. No attempt was made to determine exactly how much food coloring might be required to make the individual patient react.

Dr. James Swanson, a research associate at Toronto Children's Hospital, completed a pilot study of twelve hyperactive children in 1978. He found that nine children became hyperactive when challenged in a double-blind manner with *sufficient* amounts of dye. The children were not allowed to eat any food item which was artificially colored for four days prior to the hospital challenge. Larger, well-designed studies are presently in progress.

My awareness of the allergic-tension-fatigue syndrome

I am ashamed to admit that from 1960 to 1975 while in practice as a pediatric-allergist, I seldom recognized or diagnosed this problem. Then, as often happens in medicine, my patients taught me.

Paula

The first patient was Paula. She was five years old. Both parents had allergies. She had had typical nose, eye, and chest allergies since she was two or three years old. Her symptoms could emerge anytime during the year, not just during the warm months. In addition, her parents complained that she seemed to be unusually emotional, at times crying for hours, and she was often depressed. Paula was hyperactive, irritable, and often complained of bellyaches, diarrhea, and headaches. She could not play, learn, or adjust to school.

I examined the child, sincerely thinking she must have had brain damage at birth, but a detailed history revealed nothing to confirm my suspicion. I was perplexed, because she was exceptionally difficult to examine. I felt sorry for her parents, so instead of asking them to make their home allergy-free for two weeks, and follow that by giving Paula a multiple-food-elimination diet for the next two weeks, I asked them to do both at the same time. The child and her parents needed help for her allergies as soon as possible. In three days, her mother called to say she was extremely pleased. I assumed Paula's hay fever and asthma had improved, but her mother said no, Paula's disposition and her activity were better. I was amazed and perplexed. The mother said Paula's teacher had called to find out which "drug" the child was taking. Paula now played normally, joined in school activities and listened to stories. Relatives noted for the first time that she climbed onto their laps and liked to be kissed and cuddled. Her parents said they could now take her for a car ride. In the past, after five minutes, she was all over the car, and long auto rides were impossible. They found, for the first time, that Paula could sleep all night.

The second visit to my office, two weeks later, was a joy. Paula was pleasant, cooperative, allowed me to make a complete physical examination without objecting, and even permitted needle skin-testing without a whimper. In the next few weeks, we ascertained that milk caused irritability, hyperactivity, and throat-clearing. Corn caused diarrhea, abdominal pain, and disposition problems. Chocolate, blueberries, and mint caused hyperactivity. The smell of specific perfumes caused extreme hyperactivity within a few minutes. Paula's parents realized that these foods caused circles under her eyes, her temper to flare, and hyperactivity, crying and even a different way of talking. Three years later, Paula's school work is excellent and she has no difficulty except when she eats too much of those foods which cause her symptoms. However, small amounts are tolerated without difficulty on special occasions. She must continue to avoid certain perfumes.

Marlene

The second patient was Marlene. She was a seventeen-year-old who had received allergy-injection therapy for dust, pollen, and other common causes of allergy for several years. The referring physician asked if I would try to determine why she was so tired all the time. I candidly explained that I probably could not help her, for I still doubted that the allergic-tension-fatigue syndrome existed. Marlene lived about a hundred miles away and slept during the entire drive to Buffalo. She was admitted to the hospital for a urinary problem and was seen by me at that time. She stated she had had a headache every day of her life. She had frequent bellyaches. She often had muscle aches, especially near her back and shoulders. She said her eyes felt granular. She had no pep. On weekends she could easily sleep sixteen hours a day.

Marlene was not allowed to eat because a minor surgical procedure was scheduled the day she was admitted. The next day, she commented, she felt better. She said, in the past, she'd noted she often felt better about 11 A.M. and seemed worse again by 1:30 P.M. each day. While she was in the hospital, I requested that she drink only distilled water and eat only honey and carrots for three days. She noticed at the end of three days, she had no aches, was energetic, and felt the "best" she had in years. She was then allowed a new single food for each meal. She was told to eat only a tablespoon of the new food, then to wait at least a half hour before eating the remaining portion. She found that certain foods—potatoes, milk, and chicken—caused a headache or bellyache within half an hour; others could be eaten without difficulty. She could eat Jell-O without difficulty, but Jell-O made from water that had been used to cook potatoes caused symptoms. Three glasses of tap water caused a headache, but well water from her home or distilled or spring water caused no difficulty. (Her father had a similar problem with tap water.) During her hospital stay, it was also found that the odors of perfume, tobacco, warm plastic food trays, and cleaning solutions caused symptoms.

Her mother noted that Marlene sang songs all the way home. During the subsequent weeks, the family realized she was talkative. In contrast to her previous tendency to say little, the family complained that she talked too much. Marlene wanted to go to parties and began acting like a normal teenager. She no longer slept twelve to eighteen hours a day.

These two patients, seen within a two-week period in 1975, illustrated the two extremes of the allergic-tension-fatigue syndrome. One was a young, hyperactive child destined for many school problems. The other, older girl, suffering fatigue and constant headaches, had missed her entire opportunity for an education, as well as the fun of being a child. Why had I not believed the writings of Drs. Rowe, Randolph, Speer, and Deamer? How could I have missed it for so long? The answer is that a doctor often sees what he wants to see and is trained to see. If parents noticed their child had a better disposition, stopped wetting the bed, or seemed less tired, or less overactive after a diet, I always believed that it was because the nose and chest allergies were better.

As time passed, more and more children were observed to respond favorably to the diet that omitted certain foods and dyes. Drs. Crook and Feingold and many physicians before them appeared to be correct. Foods did, indeed, cause nervous-system symptoms associated with the allergic-tension-fatigue syndrome.

At this point I was merely beginning to learn from my patients.

Stephen

Later in 1975, I saw Stephen. He was a four-year-old, adopted, white boy who had the following problems: From the age of six months on he had had a stuffy nose all year. He had had one infection after another, especially in his ears. He'd had as many as fifteen infections in a single year. He had coughed since the age of seven months, especially when he laughed, got angry, or had a cold. He had hives and asthma by the time he was four years old. This part of the history is typical of many children who have allergies. In addition, however, his mother said that he was a nasty, violent, aggressive child. He had several temper tantrums every day. He hit his mother, punched strangers in the belly, and screamed and cried, at times for hours. He could not sleep well and was up five to six times each night. At times, he was too tired to walk and had to be carried home from a play area. He was afraid of everything. He handled everything within his reach. He tended to be extremely sad or happy at times. He vomited several times every day.

He sometimes coughed until he was exhausted. He craved milk and cheese. On one occasion, his mother tried eighteen times to make him sit down; she finally had to tie him to a chair.

He was placed on a milk-free diet. It took a full fourteen days before he improved markedly. His mother noted that he was nice to people, he stopped yelling and screaming, and he slept peacefully through the night, every night; he didn't need to nap and was not tired in the day. He seemed happy all the time and very affectionate. He stopped vomiting and coughing. He had no violent temper outbursts. In the next week or two, whenever he made a mistake and drank or ate any milk product, he became congested and was his "old" self again. Six weeks after he stopped all milk and dairy products, he had gained four pounds. His infections, ear problems, and stuffy nose stopped. He was a different child.

I decided to try to do a double-blind study to verify, scientifically, that milk bothered Stephen. It took about seven weeks to arrange for the preparation of two coded samples of "ice cream" (one made with, and one without milk), the meeting with a cameraman, the child, his parents and myself. We fed him one "ice cream," which we later determined did not contain cow's milk. Nothing happened. The next day we fed him the other coded "ice cream" made with cow's milk. Again, there was no change in his activity. I was confused and baffled. I told his mother I must have been wrong. She could feed him milk and dairy products, because milk apparently was not his problem. In about three weeks, however, I received a call that Stephen was hyperactive again. He was vomiting almost daily; his cough and earaches had returned. Milk was stopped, and he improved again. Why?

The answer was found in a book called *Food Allergy* written by Drs. Rinkel, Randolph, and Zeller (1951). They stated that if a person stops eating a food for five to twelve days, that person often will react to the food within an hour of the time it is eaten. If three or more weeks pass before the food is eaten again, there may be no bad effect. Days or weeks later, however, if the offending food continues to be eaten, it is not unusual for the original symptoms to reappear and cause trouble. Stephen's reactions could be explained.

Two years later, in 1977, his mother must still limit Stephen's milk to cooked foods. If he eats too many dairy products, his original symptoms recur. She found he could ingest more milk and dairy products during the summer months than in the winter. Dr. Rowe and Dr. Rinkel had pointed this out many years before. I find no adequate explanation for this observation.

MY SPECIAL FOOD STUDY

Although my training and background were almost entirely clinical, or directly related to the care of patients, the problem of the role of foods in hyperactivity, behavior, and learning difficulties stimulated me to attempt to do a special study related to this problem early in 1976 (Rapp 1978 b, c).

Twenty-four children, diagnosed by their pediatrician or psychologist as hyperactive, were studied. Their ages ranged from five to sixteen years. All but four of the children were presently, or had been, on at least one drug to help control their activity or behavior problems. The parents first filled in a questionnaire similar to the "Possible Common Symptoms of Allergy" questionnaire in chapter 3. This helped us quickly determine if a child had a typical allergy or the symptoms so frequently noted with the allergic-tension-fatigue syndrome.

It was found that over 70 percent had a personal history of typical allergy and 70 percent had other family members with typical allergy. In the normal population, this figure would not be above 20 percent. Over 70 percent also had symptoms, other than hyperactivity, which were typical of the allergic-tension-fatigue syndrome. Approximately 75 percent had positive skin-test reactions, indicating an allergy to pollens or dust. Parents filled in a sheet similar to the "Hyperkinesis Parent's Questionnaire" in chapter 2, so we could roughly score their child's activity level.

In an effort to see if it might be possible to predict the cause of hyperactivity, three drops of either grocery-store food coloring or liquified foods were placed under the children's tongues. We found that a well-trained allergy nurse agreed exactly with a housewife who knew little about allergy in over 80 percent of their interpretations of observations of the children's reactions. Over 80 percent of the children did not react to the control drops, either grape juice or prune juice. None of the observers, the children, or their parents were told which item was being tested. The observers found that within ten minutes, 58 percent of the children appeared to become more active from the food coloring, while about 45 percent became more active from liquified foods. Of this group, 20 percent reacted to both dyes and foods.

I then met with the parents for the first time, and placed each child on a strict one-week diet (see chapter 4 and appendix B3), which excluded food coloring, milk, wheat, eggs, cocoa, corn, and sugar in all forms. Parents recorded all foods eaten every day. At the end of the week, they scored their child's hyperactivity again to see if the score had changed. From parents' statements, it was found that over 50 percent of the children were moderately or markedly improved by the end of the week, and that the children's activity scores were much lower. Other parents felt their children were not improved and their children's activity scores remained essentially the same.

Parents were then asked to add each of the above test food items back into their child's diet, one each day. They were to watch and see if any seemed to cause a reaction. If a food appeared to cause any symptom, the parent had to confirm the food reaction by repeatedly feeding the child this food at five-day intervals to note if the food always caused the same response. From the repeated testing, it was found that 52 percent became more active from food coloring, 33 percent from sugar, 29 percent from milk, 24 percent from corn, 19 percent from cocoa, 14 percent from wheat, and 10 percent from eggs. Over 60 percent of the children reacted to more than one food or dye.

When we compared the results of tests under the tongue to the results of diet, we found that sublingual or under-the-tongue food-coloring tests seemed to be a fairly accurate way to screen patients for a food-dye sensitivity, but a *mixture* of foods (milk, wheat, eggs, cocoa, corn, and sugar) under the tongue was not reliable. Physicians knowledgeable about sublingual (under the tongue) food testing state it would have been more accurate to test separately for each food because, for example, one food may make a child tired, another hyperactive (see chapter 4).

In spite of justifiable criticism of this study, it does appear that a one-week diet omitting certain foods and food coloring did help over 50 percent of the hyperactive children, and, eighteen months later, the children who continued to avoid the offending foods continued to be significantly improved. When they made mistakes, their symptoms recurred. Over 50 percent of the children were able to discontinue Ritalin or similar drugs, although this had not been possible during previous attempts. The children not helped by diet were essentially the same eighteen months later.

One of the most startling results of the study was that many parents noticed not only that activity and behavior improved while the child was on the diet, but that other chronic complaints also dramatically subsided. These included headaches, muscle, leg, or joint aches, bellyaches or gas, nose congestion, bladder problems, and itchy skin. Some of these symptoms had been a daily problem for many years; others had been evident every week or two for a year or so. When individual foods or dyes were purposely eaten at five-day intervals, it was not unusual to find that one food item affected a child's activity, while another caused headaches, bellyaches, or other symptoms. The following is a report of one patient in this study.

Donald

Donald was an eleven-year-old, black male. As an infant, he slept poorly and cried a lot. He never napped as a young child. When his mother came to see me, she was "at the end of her rope." Teachers called every other day because of his disruptive and rude behavior. His brothers and sisters avoided him. He had no friends, was moody and always angry. He could not fall asleep at bedtime and was up and down all night to go to the bathroom. He was afraid of new situations. He tended to brag. His toe tips were cracked. He had puffy eyes. At least once a week for two or three years, he had had backaches and muscle aches. He was irritable, hyperactive, unhappy, restless, hostile, and a behavior problem. He cried frequently for no reason and talked in excess. He was not affectionate. He had been on several drugs to help control his behavior for five years. He had been on his present drug for three years, three times a day. Surprisingly, in spite of his many problems, he was an excellent student.

When Donald was skin-tested for allergies, he had a strong reaction to dust and mattress stuffing.

To evaluate the role of foods in relation to his activity and behavior problems, he was placed on a diet (see appendix B3) which omitted milk, wheat, eggs, cocoa, corn, sugar, and dyes. In twenty-four hours, he was slightly better and a week later "he had responded so dramatically that his parents could not believe it." He talked more slowly and said less, but what he said made more sense. He was more pleasant, polite, and considerate. He was not short-tempered or nervous. He didn't "fly off the handle anymore." He had no joint or muscle aches and seemed less clumsy. His nose, however, continued, occasionally, to be stuffy. (It was the grass pollen season, and he had not been treated for grass allergy.) An activity-scoring report showed a drop from 19 to 0. Sixteen weeks later, his score was only 3. Six months later his score was 2. During the week when the test foods were re-added to the diet, one at a time, he had no difficulty until he ate eggs and artificially dyed foods. His parents described these reactions as "violent." When given artificial food coloring, he talked fast, his eyes looked glassy and puffy and his face flushed. He also became stubborn, loud, and nervous, and complained of a headache. His teacher called his mother during the day to complain about his bad behavior on that day. At bedtime, his parents said he was still uncontrollable. He could not sleep.

When eggs were eaten, he became disobedient, his face flushed, his nose was stuffy, and he was so active he could not sleep. On several more occasions, at five-day intervals, his parents rechecked these foods, and each time the same symptoms appeared. To further confirm his sensitivity to these items, some unlabeled identical capsules were filled with milk and others with eggs. He quickly became active from the egg-filled capsules, but had no reactions to those filled with milk powder.

As time passed, he avoided artificial red dyes in particular. If he had symptoms, he took Alka-Seltzer Antacid Formula without Aspirin, and this helped in about twenty minutes (Randolph 1976a). He could not eat eggs in any food until he was treated with three drops of diluted egg under his tongue (see "Food Testing and Treatment" in chapter 4). If he forgot his drops, foods with eggs caused symptoms in about half an hour. If he ate too many egg-containing foods, he needed his drops twice during the day. His activity score ranged from 2 to 3 after two to four months on egg treatment. During that period he could eat eggs without difficulty for the first time. Eighteen months later, eggs continue to cause symptoms if he forgets his sublingual egg drops, but he needs the drops only twice a week. His activity score, two and one-half years after treatment, remains 3.

OTHER RECENT RESEARCH

James O'Shea, a pediatrician near Boston, completed a pilot study early in 1978, in which he studied fifteen children selected by teachers as hyperactive, with behavior and learning problems. The parents and children were interviewed weekly by a psychologist for a period of six weeks. All children were skin-tested, using a bioassay titration method (see chapter 4), for milk, wheat, egg, cocoa, corn, sugar, food coloring, apple, grape, peanut, tomato, orange, dust, mold spores, and tree pollens. Each child received sublingual (under the tongue) therapy for allergy-skin-test-positive items for a period of three weeks and for another three-week period received a placebo solution which looked and tasted identical to the allergy extract. The children received the active extract or the placebo first on a random basis. All solutions were coded in a double-blind manner by a pharmacist. During the study the children were allowed to ingest all foods in moderation except preservatives and food additives. Parents kept daily diet records.

He found that seven of the children had a positive family history of allergy, ten had a personal history of allergy, and eleven had typical physical signs of respiratory allergy. When the code was broken it was found that about 79 percent of the parents and 57 percent of the teachers could readily differentiate the period when the children received food therapy, in contrast to the placebo.

L. B., a thirteen-year-old white male, participated in this study. He happened to receive the placebo solution during the first three-week period and little change was noted in the child by his teacher, parents or the psychologist. During the second three weeks, however, when he was receiving sublingual food therapy, his mother commented as follows: He was the best he had been in years. He was unbelievably calmer. For the first time since the age of seven months, he slept through the night and was much less restless. He did not lose his temper once. He sat through the *entire* supper period and sat quietly in the evening for the first time in his life. He discussed his feelings sensibly. He was able to nap. He didn't beat up his sisters. He was less sensitive and seemed less depressed and fearful. He read an entire book in one week. His teachers commented that he volunteered more in class and was doing assigned work on time, as well as unassigned work. He was definitely more conscientious in all aspects.

His attitude was less sullen. Outside the classroom he was still active, but not punching, hitting, and insolent as before.

On several occasions his mother noted that after the ingestion of certain foods he would have a marked change in personality. After red dyes he had a "crying jag and deep depression." After chocolate pudding he was "literally flying." After colored chewing gum, he threw a brick at a friend. On a few occasions, his mother forgot to give him his sublingual drops and his nose became stuffy and his behavior and activity became noticeably worse.

In 1978 Trites and his associates in Ottawa, Ontario, reported the results of part of an ongoing study which included the evaluation of the role of foods in hyperactivity in children. He found that approximately two-thirds of the children studied had an elevated antibody called IgE to one or more of forty-two foods tested by the radioallergosorbent test (RAST). All children were placed on a diet which excluded their individual RAST-positive foods for a three-week period and their activity and behavior was compared to a similar period when they ate foods which were RAST-negative. The patients were unaware which diet they were receiving during the six-week period. Trites found that 20 percent of the hyperactive children studied were improved significantly during the diet which excluded potentially allergenic RAST-positive foods. When children accidentally ate some RAST-positive foods, reactions were often noted within a short period of time.

Since early in this century, food sensitivities have been suspected as the cause not only of hyperactivity, but also of many other chronic complaints affecting many areas of the body (Hoobler 1916, Cooke 1922, Randolph 1947, Rowe 1950). Due to lack of scientific documentation which stringently follows today's standards, some physicians continue to doubt that foods can adversely affect many aspects of a patient's health. Current acceptable, but inconclusive, research is now "suggesting" that artificial food coloring does indeed alter the activity and behavior of some children. In time, it is anticipated that proof will be available to document that not only food coloring, but also many foods or other exposures in our environment can cause deleterious health problems in many age groups (Rea 1976, 1977, 1978, Miller 1972, 1977).

2 · Questions Most Parents Ask about Hyperactivity, Behavior and Learning Problems

This chapter simply explains the common terms used in relation to hyperactivity (or fatigue) and learning problems. The scope of the problem, common methods of treatment, drugs, and special challenges confronting parents are discussed. Tips are given to help parents cope more effectively.

What is hyperactivity?

Unfortunately, there is no simple definition. In contrast to normally active children, hyperactive youngsters cannot complete a chore, sit through a meal, watch an entire television program, or listen to the end of a story. They are often in perpetual motion, unable to sit without wiggling, moving, or fidgeting. They're often clumsy. They don't accept discipline. They may cry, complain, and seem depressed or angry. There is, however, a wide range of normal activity which can vary with the age of the child and circumstances. For example, the activity of a toddler has exhausted many a mother. It is normally a period filled with boundless energy. Some parents complain, however, that their infant or child is very active, only to be reassured that no problem exists. The physician may be incorrect because the child's activity appears normal during the short period of the examination, even though the child may be excessively active at home. It is not unusual for mothers, in particular, to feel extremely guilty because they have been made to believe their child's inability to rest and relax is in some way their fault. They sometimes stop mentioning the problem because no one listens. When the child starts school, the teacher confirms their suspicions. When someone knowledgeable, such as a teacher, observes a child for several hours regularly, it's easy to compare activity levels and select youngsters who repeatedly disrupt the class and can't function normally.

Other parents believe all children act similarly to their youngster and don't believe the physician when he suggests their child appears overactive. Parents often state that he's "just being a boy" or that the whole family acts this way. If both your physician and the teacher agree your child is hyperactive, believe them. They are probably correct. If both you and the teacher believe your child is hyperactive, give your physician more details. With more information, he, also, may agree and provide essential help and guidance.

What is the difference between hyperactivity and hyperkinesis?

Some people use these terms interchangeably, but hyperactivity is only one part of hyperkinesis. The latter term includes the inability to concentrate on one thing, or a short attention span; a rush to do everything, or impulsiveness; flitting from thing to thing, or easy distractibility.

Which characteristics are common in hyperkinetic children?

Hyperkinetic children may have many of the following problems, on occasion or all the time:
Can't sit still
    To watch television
    To hear a story to the end
    To ride in a car
    To eat an entire meal
Can't concentrate
    To complete a chore
    To study in school
    To understand discipline
    To play a game
Can't control emotions
    Cry easily and often
    Fight often and readily
    Are aggressive and bully
    Are depressed
    Have temper tantrums and emotional outbursts
    Fall apart with criticism

Don't speak normally
    Speak too loudly
    Speak too much
    Babble and not make sense
    Have sudden speech outbursts
    Stutter or lisp
    Interrupt conversations
    Seem "spaced out" at times
Have poor dispositions
    Are irritable
    Are unhappy
    Fight with other children
    Have few friends
    Become frustrated easily
May hurt themselves or others
    Appear clumsy or awkward
    Run too fast
    Bump into walls and furniture
    Bite or hit other children or adults
    Are impulsive without thinking
May break things
    Handle or finger everything near them
    Damage touched items accidentally
Aren't normally affectionate
    Resist sitting on parents' laps
    Dislike being cuddled
    Dislike being kissed and hugged
Can't sleep properly
    Have difficulty getting to sleep
    Are unable to stay asleep (babies included)
    Roll and toss all night
    Have nightmares and bad dreams
    Cry out in sleep
    Sleep with clenched fists, stiff arms and legs
    Awaken irritable, tired, not refreshed
May not like themselves
    Call themselves stupid
    Think others don't like them
    Dislike themselves and have a poor self-image
    Are depressed at times
    Say life isn't worth the effort

What is a specific learning disability (SLD)?

Children with this problem may not speak or write properly for many reasons. Each child may have a specific problem with one or more of the following: listening, thinking, talking, reading, writing, spelling, or arithmetic. Each individual problem can be complex and complicated. For example, a listening problem in an SLD is not due to a malfunction of the ear causing some degree of deafness. SLD children may hear the words but may be unable to recognize, interpret, or visualize what is being said. Some may hear and understand *only* when they can see the words being spoken. Translating what is heard into words can be another problem. Auditory perception can sometimes be improved by having a child shut his eyes and listen to a bouncing ball, a bell, or some other common sound. Visual perception may be helped by hitting a Ping-Pong ball or working with puzzles which are three dimensional. Specially trained teachers knowledgeable in this area can be most helpful in guiding parents who want to help teach their child how to increase his perceptual skills.

Included in SLD would be problems associated with minimal brain dysfunction. Not included in SLD would be problems due to vision or sight, hearing (deafness), coordination, mental retardation, emotional problems or stressful family situations.

What is meant by minimal brain dysfunction (MBD)?

Children who have both hyperactivity and learning disabilities are considered to have minimal brain dysfunction. The definition does not include children who have only hyperactivity or only learning disabilities. MBD children may have very mild or very severe problems and may have associated behavior difficulties. The problems with MBD children may be subtle, not immediately obvious, as in youngsters who have cerebral palsy or severe brain damage. *Cerebral* and *brain dysfunction* are terms which mean essentially the same as minimal brain dysfunction.

What characteristics do MBD children have?

Short Attention Span. These children need activities which require change and movement. They can't sit and read quietly for hours or even watch their favorite television program without wiggling or movement.

Easy Distractibility. If all is quiet and calm, a child may be all right, but in a room filled with exciting things or people, control is completely lost.

Overactivity. The activity is disorganized, not just moving, but moving aimlessly. These children expend lots of energy to accomplish nothing. Some may appear perfectly normal on a one-to-one basis; for example, in a physician's office, but not in a schoolroom or an active household. They can't control their urge to move or wiggle.

Impulsiveness. MBD children often can't hold back. They blurt out whatever they are thinking. They suddenly move or jump before they should, often hurting themselves. They can't stand to wait in line or take their turn. They touch the forbidden. They do things so fast, they don't have time to think. They need action.

Emotional Problems. They just can't control their emotions. They cry easily, anger easily, and laugh easily. At times they explode. Temper tantrums may be extreme and often. They don't try to be bad, they just can't control themselves.

Discipline Problems. Some can't concentrate long enough to hear what they've done wrong. They may repeat a mistake shortly after they are corrected. Spanking is often useless.

Poor Coordination. Sometimes big movements or gross motor coordination, such as running, is a problem, but more often they have trouble doing little things with their hands and fingers or with what is called fine motor coordination. They can't tie their shoes or fold a piece of paper exactly in half. Speaking may be a problem, because the tongue does not always move normally. Affected children often talk too loudly, too much, and may not speak sensibly. Such children move unrelated parts of their body when it is not necessary. For example, the left hand moves when the right hand is writing. The mouth moves as the child taps his fingers. Part of the coordination problem is noted in judging distance. Some children run so fast and hard that they can't stop before they bump into walls and furniture. They fall and hurt themselves because their arms or legs try to go too far, too fast. These children may batter themselves. See chapter 5.

Perception Problems. This means children have trouble telling "left" from "right," "in front of" from "in back of," or "before" from "after." The many fine details of writing the alphabet correctly or doing arithmetic are often overwhelming for affected youngsters.

Learning Problems Related to Reading and Spelling. Children with this type of problem often speak words and sentences later than normal children. When they try to read, their mind flits so fast they can't remember the first letter of a word by the time they are looking at the last letter. They tend to guess. The problems are compounded or made worse by the inability to concentrate for a long time, and by their impulsiveness, rushing to get going, and easy distractibility, which causes the children to go off on tangents whenever something distracts them.

What is meant by minimal brain damage?

This term means the brain has actually been damaged in some manner: at birth, by infection, a poison, a toxin, or accidental injury. This term should not be used if someone means minimal brain dysfunction, for this means the brain only has difficulty functioning at peak performance, it is not damaged. If your hand is caught in the door of a car, it is damaged. If your fingers are so poorly coordinated that you can't play the piano, the hand is not damaged but there is some dysfunction or difficulty in doing something which requires a large amount of coordination.

What is fatigue?

Some children are not hyperactive, but too tired. They sleep longer than other children and cannot get through the day without naps. They may stop in the middle of play to rest. These children sleep during car rides or after eating. They may be too tired to join in normal activities with other children. At times, their activity ranges from nil to extreme hyperactivity, on and off, all day or some days (Randolph 1947, Rowe 1950, 1959, Crook 1961).

Is hyperactivity increasing?

Exact figures are not known, but the general impression is that there are more overactive children in classrooms than ever before. It is estimated that there are between four and five million children in the United States with hyperactivity and learning disabilities. A large number of these children use drugs on a regular basis to help modify their activity. Teachers who have taught for over twenty years state the problem is definitely more evident now than ever before. Increased awareness accounts for only part of the apparent rise. We cannot explain why the problem is more evident in certain geographic areas than in others. Dr. Feingold, in his book, states that over 25 percent of children in some areas of California and New York have a hyperkinetic learning disability.

Is hyperactivity outgrown?

Many infants or children appear to become less hyperactive as they grow up. Sometimes this requires months, at times years. Some children, however, grow into hyperactive adults. Maturity makes it easier for hyperactive children to control their activity or channel it into a socially acceptable form, such as into sports activities or working in a hectic, active business. Long-term studies of hyperactive children through teenage years indicate that affected children often have persistent problems adjusting at home, at work or school, and socially (Menkes et al. 1967, Mendelson et al. 1971).

What causes hyperactivity, fatigue, and behavior and learning problems?

These are each a mixed bag (Brutten et al. 1973, Levy 1973). In general, there are many causes for each of these problems. In each child, there is often one or more reasons for the symptoms. Each child must be considered separately. In some patients, a specific cause may not be found. Possible common causes include the following:

· Certain medical problems such as anemia, hypothyroidism, hypoglycemia, lead poisoning, sickle cell anemia or disease, intestinal parasites, visual or hearing problems, and mental illness.

· Damage to a child's nervous system before or at the time of birth. Damage can occur later due to illnesses, such as infections within the brain (bacterial meningitis or viral encephalitis) or due to accidents or injuries involving the brain or skull.

· Allergies in the form of the allergic-tension-fatigue syndrome (see chapter 1). At present, this causative factor is seldom recognized or diagnosed by many physicians. If this is the cause of your child's problem, it may be possible to treat it easily and quickly (see Randolph 1947, Kittler and Baldwin 1970, Millman et al. 1976, Rapaport and Flint 1976, Roth 1978, Trites et al. 1978).

· Psychological or social problems often arise in children who live in disrupted homes.

· Hereditary or genetic problems. Close or distant relatives may have similar problems.

There is no doubt that a deficiency of certain vitamin or mineral supplements may contribute to nervous system problems. Scientific documentation is not available at the present time to state how many children with MBD or hyperactivity have these types of deficiencies (Hoffer 1974; see "The Vitamin Controversy" in chapter 4).

Can infants be hyperactive?

They can. Most babies sleep twelve or more hours per day. A hyperactive child may sleep for an hour or an hour and a half and then fret and cry for the next six or eight hours. This will strain the baby, mother, marriage, and the baby's physician. New mothers often feel guilty because they think or have been told the problem is their fault. They are told they are nervous and this in turn causes their baby to be nervous. How can a mother not be nervous, tired, and bewildered if a new baby sleeps such a little while?

Formula or diet changes may relieve the problem if, in particular, milk, sugar (dextrose), corn, soy, or cereals are at fault. The inability to sleep through the night or nap may be a persistent problem for years in some food sensitive children until the proper diagnosis is made.

All infant restlessness is not due to foods. If your physician cannot determine why your baby can't sleep, a thorough evaluation in a hospital may be necessary.

Can breast feeding result in hyperactivity?

Yes. Although breast feeding is surely the best method to feed a baby, food proteins pass through the breast milk which make some babies restless. A nursing mother can put herself on the rotary diet in chapter 3 for a week or two to see if the baby seems better. As individual foods are again eaten by the mother, she can notice the effect each food has on her baby, as well as on herself. If the baby also eats some foods, the foods must be selected from the identical daily rotary diet list used by the mother.

Many breast-fed babies are given supplementary bottles of sugar water and various kinds of milk or other foods. Any of these can cause increased activity in some infants.

Can a parent easily tell an overactive child from a normal active toddler?

No. This may be a trying period for any parent or child. Bursts of activity are common for children aged two to four years. Right from wrong must be taught and learned. The easiest way to come to the correct conclusion is to observe your child in groups of children the same age. Does your child stand out? Is your child's behavior repeatedly disruptive at parties, at church, or at family and social gatherings?

Can cow's milk cause hyperactivity or other problems in infancy or later on?

Some infants remain hyperactive until their cow's-milk formula is switched to soybean milk or juice. Although most infants improve in a few days, some might not seem better for about two weeks (Kittler and Baldwin 1970, Dohan and Grasberger 1973).

A more common problem associated with drinking milk in infants and adults is a lactose intolerance which causes bellyaches, bloating, and diarrhea (Oski 1977). Milk contains an undigestible sugar called lactose which is broken down into digestible simple sugars in the small intestine by an enzyme called lactase. Occasionally, babies are born without lactase and have feeding problems shortly after birth. Infection in the intestines or the use of antibiotics at any age can cause a temporary loss of lactase and associated intestinal problems when milk is ingested. People naturally lose their lactase as they become older, so adults often can't drink a glass of milk without abdominal discomfort. Sixty to 100 percent of Eskimos, American Indians, Africans, and Asiatics lack lactase, while only about 25 percent of white Americans have this problem.

If you or your family normally drink milk, but you would like to find out if you have a milk problem, try not drinking milk or eating any product which contains milk (see appendix B5) for a full five days. Then drink two glasses of cold milk on an empty stomach. If problems arise, check with your physician. Special tests can be done to confirm if you lack lactase. If you do, your physician may recommend that you avoid milk, add a commercial lactase to the milk you drink, or drink acidophilus milk to help restore your normal intestinal bacterial flora.

It has been observed, but not scientifically documented, that enzyme deficiencies may subside after proper therapy for food or chemical sensitivities (see chapter 4). More research is needed in this area (Buisseret 1978, Rapp 1978a).

Are you always making excuses for your child's behavior?

It is natural for parents to blame others for their child's difficulties—at first. But if you find you are always taking your active child's side against neighbors, your other children, teachers, and relatives, it may not be a series of unfortunate misunderstandings or bad luck. It may not be a stage he is going through; face up to it, your child may be different and his problems may be a flag of distress indicating a desperate need for help.

Do people disagree about your child?

It would not be unusual if they did. Mothers often recognize overactivity or behavior problems before fathers. They are home with the child for longer periods of time. Parents may recognize a problem long before relatives or your physician is aware of, or acknowledges, it. A physician sees a child in a one-to-one situation, for only a few minutes, and some children may be able to show excellent control for short periods of time.

The kindergarten or nursery-school teacher can recognize a problem hyperactive child very quickly. If foods are factors, the activity may become most evident after a morning snack or lunch. Once a child takes a drug, such as Ritalin, each morning, the morning teacher may see a normal child, while the afternoon teacher sees a child with a problem. If a child has a chance to run about in gym, he may be less active during the next period. If he has to sit quietly, read, or do math, he may quickly reveal his inability to control himself. If a food causes an undesirable effect six to eight hours after it is eaten, your child's teacher may never notice any unusual symptoms. The symptom would be evident only after school hours.

Are hyperactive children harder to raise?

Yes. Hyperactive children can be trying and exasperating, even though they are loved. They may be a constant or intermittent problem, even a daily challenge or threat. They disrupt the entire household. This leads to guilt, and parents wonder why they are upset not only with the child, but with their own feelings. Is it their fault? What did they do wrong? Often it is not the parents' fault in any way. They have done their best and only by learning more about the problem can they hope to handle their individual child's special needs and possibly help him to become the lovable child they know he can be (Stewart and Olds 1973, Brutten et al. 1973, Levy 1973).

To complicate and compound the situation, hyperactive children often don't like themselves. They realize they have few friends and have a poor self-image. Everyone seems to criticize and dislike them. They realize they have a problem and they wonder why. They may dislike how they act and feel. In an effort to feel important or outstanding, some may engage in antisocial activity or behavior. A parent's love is essential to help keep such children on the correct path.

Are parents of hyperactive children themselves hyperactive?

One or both may be. All parents are not calm, quiet, and low key. Some families are active, alert, and always in motion. Their children are more apt to be active than those in a placid family. It is possible that this family trait is a bit exaggerated in one child. Grandparents may recall if parents were hyperactive as children. With time and maturity, overactive children almost always become less active adults. It is also certainly possible that a food which is making the child hyperactive, is also making a parent more active than "normal" (Morrison and Stewart 1971).

Should you wait for your child to outgrow the problem?

It depends on how severe the problem is. If the child is impossible—you can't wait. Can he cope at home, at school, and with friends? If the answer is no, he needs help—now. If you wait, the problems may mushroom. The child will not like himself or others because he is not liked. If he can't sit in school and concentrate, he can't learn. The longer he doesn't keep up, the more difficult it will be to catch up later on. He may develop defensive habit patterns which are hard to break. He may develop a bad reputation which will require much "good" to eliminate. Your child must conform to an acceptable minimum or he can become a most unhappy, frustrated child, teenager, and adult (Menkes et al. 1967, Mendelson and Stewart 1971).

Are hyperactives bright?

Surprisingly, in spite of severe activity problems, some children do very well in school. The majority of hyperactive children, however, in spite of average or above-average intelligence, are unable to work at their full potential. They have a good brain, but their nervous system is too sensitive. Their motor is racing when it should be on "idle." They often have active imaginations which lead to innovative or ingenious ways to create bedlam and havoc. They can't concentrate long enough to hear the teacher's instructions, let alone to try to carry them out. The room seems to be full of distracting sights, sounds, things to touch, and odors (Rapaport and Flint 1976, Miller, 1977).

Does discipline help?

The hyperactive child can't concentrate long enough to hear what he has done wrong or how to correct his behavior. Physical punishment or spanking may only relieve your anxieties and hurt your hand. Such children may not mean to be bad. Much of their difficulty is due to their uncontrollable urge to wiggle or move about. This, in itself, leads to a greater chance of accidents involving the child and the family's possessions. Dr. Robert Buckley (1972), a California psychiatrist, has stated that affected children may have a reduced response to pain, so fearless foolishness can be a problem.

What should you do when your hyperactive misbehaves?

Should you make excuses because he is hyperactive? Should you attempt to treat him like your other children? Should you walk away so you do not spank him too hard? There are no easy answers. Your physician will help to guide you between reasonable and unreasonable parental behavior. Don't expect yourself to be perfect. Try to set reasonable limits and make exceptions when it is sensible to do so. Expect your child, however, to try harder. He can control himself to a degree and this must be fostered and encouraged. With strong motivation, he may be able to do better. He may be able to watch his favorite television cartoon with less difficulty than he can sit through dinner. He may be better at the doctor's office than at home. He is the same at both times, but his motivation is different. Remember, don't make your child feel that he is bad or a failure. He is well aware of his faults. Stress that you love him and know he did not want to do something wrong. Let him know that he is forgiven, but that he must try much harder to be good.

If you are going to try discipline, don't do it when he is so wound-up that he barely notices his punishment. Try to wait until he is more quiet, explain what he did wrong and why you must try to help him learn by using discipline. If such an approach does not help, talk to your family physician.

Does nonspecific treatment help hyperactive children?

If children are hyperactive, they tend to be very sensitive to change and responsive to stimuli. Such children are easily distracted by noise, sound, light, and movement. Obviously, one help is to reduce external stimuli by making your home a more quiet, restful place. Angie Nall, a former teacher, has a homelike hospital for learning-disabled children in Beaumont, Texas. She finds that no radio or television, speaking in a slow, quiet voice, and keeping the environment calm and relaxed is very helpful. The atmosphere is one of love and care, but it is firm and controlled. If your home is like a game room at the fair, your child doesn't stand a chance.

How can teachers help your child?

If your child cannot function in a regular classroom, ask about the available alternatives in your area. Are there special classes or schools or clinics? Try to have your child placed in an area such as a cubicle, which is less distracting. A seat near a door or window may be too stimulating. If too many things, knick-knacks, etc., are sitting around in a room, there is simply too much to excite a hyperactive child. Teachers also can set priorities and determine what is important for a child to learn. Limits must be set and adhered to consistently. Rewards and genuine concern, love and interest will help motivate a child to try harder. Most children truly want to please their parents and teachers. They want to be liked and accepted. Try to emphasize the positive.

How are hyperactivity-learning disorders treated?

The usual methods include one or more of the following:
· Drugs to make children calm down.
· Special teaching, either in a regular or smaller class. Specific help in certain subjects part-time in a resource room, while spending the rest of the time in regular classes, may help some children cope and learn better. Private tutoring is needed only for special problem children who live in areas where other therapy is not readily available. Although many hyperactive children have poor coordination, they can improve their ability with special lessons or training. If they play ball better, they are more apt to be accepted rather than ridiculed by their playmates and they will have more reasons to like themselves.
· Help from a school or other psychologist. Many MBD or hyperactive children need a psychological evaluation.
· Help for the family. Counseling is needed to teach parents and siblings how to cope and understand. In general, MBD or hyperactive children need a routine at home, so the same things are done at about the same time each day. Getting up, breakfast, lunch, dinner, going to bed, television, and play should be routine. Decrease surprise and variations. If the unexpected happens, try to spend a few moments quietly explaining and preparing your child for the change. Keep things going as smoothly as possible. The family also needs help with discipline, how and when to do it, and what to expect and not expect from the affected child and the other children. Your other children may need some explanation so they don't think they are causing your hyperactive child's problem. They may be afraid that they also will become hyperactive. Or they may be envious of the attention your problem child receives.
· Although this is not usually considered, hyperactive children should be seen by an allergist or ecologist (see appendix C3) who believes, and is successful, in determining which foods (or other items) cause activity and learning problems. In the meantime, start to observe if your child suddenly gets wound up after he eats certain foods such as sugar or chocolate, or colored items. Is he worse after eating? You may not have noticed it.

What are some no-no's?

Don't tell your child everything he has done wrong. Emphasize the things he has done right. On these occasions reward him or tell him he is wonderful, right away. Remember, he can't concentrate for very long and he may forget what he did right. He'll try harder and like himself better if you love and reward him.

Don't try to change all your child's bad tendencies at one time. He can't comply. Pick on one small aggravation and encourage him to correct that one thing. When he's better with that, praise him and go on to another small thing.

Don't say one thing one day and something different the next. Both parents must agree and make consistent rules and stick to them. Be firm and specific. For example, don't tolerate too many interruptions or embarrassing public outbursts. Let him know exactly what he can and cannot do.

Don't expect him to make decisions. Decide for him, but give him a voice in the major ones. This is easily accomplished by offering choices. You narrow the possibilities to two or three which are acceptable, then the final selection is made from these: no discussing and no fussing.

Don't avoid letting him do anything because he always does everything wrong. Pick a little chore and give it to him as an assignment. He needs some self-esteem in order to feel needed and wanted.

Don't try to do everything for him because you can do it faster and better. The entire family must learn to be patient. It will take him a little longer, but he must do it for himself.

Don't ask him to do something that is impossible. Select chores he can do. Handling your best china is not for him.

Don't shout, scream, talk through your teeth, or threaten. Try a calm, relaxed voice which doesn't sound mad or irritated. Speak slowly and in a low voice. Smile. It will work wonders—for you and your child.

Don't complain about everything. Expect a little breakage. He will be slow and he will be disorganized. Don't expect him to remember several things at once. Don't get uptight about little things. It's bad for you and for him.

Give your child checklists. It makes it easier. He doesn't have to remember so much.

Don't embarrass your child in front of his friends by telling him he's acting up again and needs another pill.

Don't pick a time when the house is hectic and he is not paying attention to give him directions. Even if you do it slowly and carefully, there may be too much going on for him to hear or do.

Don't assume he understands. After you have explained what has to be done, see if he can tell you what he is to do.

Don't try to be your child's teacher. It's a hard role to fill. Let those trained in that area work with him. You have more than enough to do being a parent.

You can use physical punishment, but don't get carried away. Don't continue a punishment for two weeks; he won't remember why he's being punished for that long. Even if you only wait until dad gets home, your child may have forgotten what he did wrong.

Don't reject your child; he's yours, for better or for worse. If he knows you sometimes get very upset with him, but still love him, it makes it much easier for him to like himself. He must like himself. When you become frustrated and discouraged with his behavior, he knows it. A disgusted look or a slight irritation in your voice is recognized and merely adds to the problem.

Don't assume that something he eats can or cannot cause his behavior or activity problems because some physician or person told you so. You be the judge. Watch your child. If he is fine and suddenly gets wild after he eats, drinks, gets near or smells something, pay attention. If this happens repeatedly, you may have an answer (see chapter 4). There may be a fast, easy way to help your child.

Where do you go for help if your child is hyperactive?

Talk to your physician first. He may help you or suggest that you see a specialist who cares for hyperactive children. Both parents should be present for the visit; one detail concerning the birth and early development of your child may hold the hidden clue to the present problem. Talk to your child's teacher and school counselor or psychologist. Many areas have local organizations that have regular meetings to discuss various aspects of learning problems. These groups may give you more insight about avenues for possible help (see appendix C2).

If you or your physician believe allergy may be a factor, read chapter 3. If you have a nail in your shoe which causes your foot to be sore, the cure is easy. Take out the nail. Putting ointments on the foot doesn't solve the problem. If your child is acting different when he eats certain food, don't make him take drugs—stop him from eating the food that causes his abnormal behavior.

How do you find the right person to help your child?

Trial and error. Find a physician who understands and seems successful in handling children with problems similar to your child's. If a teacher feels your child is merely spoiled and needs discipline, ask yourself, Is he? If he definitely is not, try another teacher. What the teacher says may be true to a degree, but some teachers are specially trained or, by nature, have more understanding and success with such children than others. Seek out this type of teacher if you can. Sometimes merely changing schools will solve the problem.

Will the doctor order more tests?

He may. Sometimes a brain wave or electroencephalogram, called an EEG, is ordered. This EEG may sometimes provide a clue which explains your child's inattention, staring spells, or twitches. In some children, brain waves may become normal when offending foods are omitted from a child's diet.

Will other doctors be needed?

Sometimes a child may need a complete eye examination by an ophthalmologist, ear or hearing tests from an otologist, psychological testing from a school or other psychologist (rarely a psychiatrist), a thorough nervous-system study by a neurologist, or an allergy evaluation from an allergist. Your family physician or pediatrician will try to guide you to the type of physician whom he feels will be most helpful for your child. Some communities have inexpensive hospital or other clinics to help with counseling and psychological evaluations.

What will the hyperactivity specialist do?

After asking you to fill in a detailed form and to discuss your child's history, the hyperactivity specialist will give the child a thorough physical examination. As mentioned before, hyperactivity is a mixed bag. Many things can cause this type of difficulty and the doctor will try to discover the basis of your child's problem and recommend appropriate treatment. Don't be disappointed if your child is found to be physically normal; be relieved. Special tests for the nervous system, however, may show some slight variations, often called "soft" neurological signs.

What are "soft" neurological signs?

This means that the "usual" examination by the neurologist or nervous system specialist shows nothing abnormal. "Soft" signs include little things which indicate that a child is not as well coordinated for his age as most children. For example, he may have trouble writing d's or b's. He may have to erase often because he has trouble making small loops or circles when he writes letters. He may reverse letters and write "saw" instead of "was." He may be unable to hop on one foot or skip rope. He can't easily and quickly touch his thumb to his second, third, fourth, and fifth fingers. He gets right and left mixed up. For example, he has difficulty putting his left hand on his right ear. He may have trouble turning his head to the left without turning his body, or looking to the right without moving his head. These are little things, but they show a physician a child has a slight weakness in his central nervous system.

DRUGS USED TO TREAT THIS PROBLEM

Commercial Name	**Chemical or Generic Name**
Ritalin	methylphenidate HCL
Atarax or Vistaril	hydroxyzine HCL
Benadryl	diphenhydramine HCL
Dexedrine	dextroamphetamine
Mellaril	thioridazine HCL
Cylert	pemoline
Thorazine	chlorpromazine
Tofranil	imipramine HCL

Why do amphetamines quiet a hyperactive child?

We don't really know. We do know that amphetamines, such as Benzedrine, make most people jumpy and nervous. Why hyperactive children become less active is a puzzle. There are many theories. One theory is that although the children are physically hyperactive in that they move about more than normal, they are physiologically underactive. By that, I mean there is some evidence to show that they have less reactive brainwaves, less reactive skin changes, slower heart rate, and less reactive responses to stress. It is thought that amphetamines may alter certain brain enzymes, such as serotonin, norepinephrine, and especially dopamine, so physiologic underactivity becomes more normal and overactivity stops (Buckley 1972, Wender 1973).

Any tips regarding Ritalin?

Some detailed information about Ritalin might be helpful because this drug is a commonly prescribed medicine to alter the activity and behavior of children. Many children respond favorably two to three days after the drug is started. It must be given when the stomach is empty. Try to schedule the dose about thirty to forty-five minutes before eating. The medicine helps for about four hours.

It is best to give it at the same time each day. For example, at 7:00 A.M. and again at 11:00 to 11:30 A.M. Give a dose after school and again before bed, if it is needed that often.

Ritalin can safely be used with some medicines, such as aspirin or antibiotics, but check with your physician to be entirely sure.

It should be given regularly if it helps, and some physicians believe it should not be stopped on weekends or during the summer months. Some recent research indicated that if children learn when they are taking the drug, they continue to learn best if they use the drug regularly (Swanson et al. 1976). More studies to verify this are needed.

How does a physician decide which drug to use?

He selects the drug from experience, based upon your child's history and physical examination. Most physicians have personal preferences due to their experience using certain drugs. Regardless of which drug he selects, the drug is used initially only on a "trial" basis. If the drug helps, the dose will be adjusted so the most "good" and the least "bad" is noticed when it is used.

When a physician selects any drug, he considers the pros and cons carefully. Will not giving the drug, in the long run, be more harmful than giving it? In general, untreated hyperactivity is more of a problem than the drugs used to treat it. This, however, is not always true, and the final decision rests with the effect the drug has upon your child. If it does not help activity (or behavior) or it causes undesirable side-effects, other drugs may be tried. It is not uncommon for some children to try several drugs before one is found which helps. Sometimes, no drugs seem to relieve a patient's symptoms.

How do these drugs affect your child?

In general, if the medication helps, it means that your child slows down enough so he can concentrate for longer periods of time, but not so much that he is a zombie. His basic personality is usually not altered, although he would be less exuberant. Sometimes, these drugs alter behavior and make the child act better, but the activity problem persists. All children are not the same, and what helps some children, may not help others.

Parents can tell when their child needs more medication, but often the child is not able to recognize that he is "out of control." Help your doctor and child by keeping a record of what happens to your child when he is taking a drug.

Relay the valuable observations of your child's teacher to your physician. Everyone must be communicating. Your physician needs your help to determine what is best for your child.

What are the undesirable side effects of drugs used to treat hyperactivity?

Common ones include loss of appetite, dizziness, inability to sleep well, headaches, and loss of mental alertness. Some complain of nausea or an upset stomach, diarrhea or a dry mouth.

Sometimes symptoms are noted only when the drugs are first started; in other children problems appear only after the drugs are used for long periods of time. Drugs which cause a loss of appetite over a long period of time may interfere with a child's normal growth. Weigh your child once a month if you are concerned and show your records to your child's physician.

Uncommon possible side effects of some drugs used to modify activity include rashes, irritability, depression, hives, joint pain, rapid heart beat, shakiness, swollen saliva glands, blurred vision, changes in blood pressure, jaundice, and confusion.

Are these drugs dangerous?

The bad reactions listed above can occur. This does not mean that they will occur. They are listed not to frighten you, but to help you watch your child so that if any of these problems do arise, you can check with your physician. Many children on these drugs notice only slight drowsiness or loss of appetite. If any drug is taken in an overdose, it can be harmful. Be sure the child does not take his own medication. Keep all drug bottles in a locked medicine chest if your child is a toddler. At school, be sure only the nurse or teacher gives your child medication.

Addiction is not a problem. Using a prescribed drug is not drug abuse. It may be a necessity, unless you can determine the cause of the problem and eliminate it.

If your child is using activity-modifying drugs, a physician should be consulted at regular intervals to be certain that the drug is still needed and that it is helpful. Many children seem to need less or no medicine on weekends or during the summer months when their activity does not need to be restricted. Even if a drug cannot be stopped, maybe the dose needs to be lowered (see above "Any Tips Regarding Ritalin?").

How can medication be given at school?

You will need a note from your physician stating when your child should receive medicine. In most schools, the school nurse or the child's teacher will give him the medicine. In many states, children cannot carry their own medicines in their pockets, purses, or lunch boxes.

Older children, in particular, are often embarrassed to take medicine, so discretion and thoughtfulness should be followed, and the drug given to the child in private. If problems arise, try to have the teacher or school official talk with your physician. Discussing a problem often solves it.

Are different types of diets recommended for hyperactive children?

In chapter 4 of this book, a diet omitting food coloring, milk, wheat, eggs, cocoa, corn, and sugar is suggested to determine if the child improves. If your child is better, the section "How to Do the

Diet" explains how to determine which suspect foods might cause your child's difficulty.

Dr. Ben Feingold (see appendix B16) recommends a diet that omits artificial food coloring, artificial flavoring, and natural salicylates.

Dr. William Crook (see appendix B18) in Tennessee suggests a rare food diet which is low in carbohydrates and food additives. He also recommends vitamin B complex and vitamin C.

When children improve, do their problems go away?

No. Most children have developed habit patterns and continue to react in an undesirable way to certain situations. They are not only conditioned, but almost expected to react badly. Once they are better, their responses gradually change. It requires a little time to learn new, acceptable responses. Counseling may be necessary and prove helpful at this time.

Occasionally a child improves remarkably at home, but the teacher notices no change. Once a child has been a particularly difficult pupil, the teacher may have been justifiably conditioned to constantly watch, suspect, and even accuse. She knows this child is a source of disruption. The teacher sometimes cannot recognize that a child's behavior has changed. The pattern at school continues to deteriorate, while at home, the child is much better. The problem is sometimes solved by changing the child to a different classroom or school. A new teacher has no preconceived impressions about the child and can evaluate him as he is, not as he had been.

Sometimes, the teacher is correct. The child is overactive in school because of a food, contact, or odor to which the child is not exposed at home. A mother may determine the cause by talking to the teacher or observing her child in school.

Is your child hyperactive?

Try filling out the "Hyperkinesis Parent's Questionnaire." See what your child's score is now and compare that to his score later on. Before reading further, do the test.

How do you interpret the score?

The purpose of the score is solely for comparison. It will enable you to tell if your child is remaining the same or becoming better or worse.

THE HYPERKINESIS PARENT'S QUESTIONNAIRE

Please answer all questions. Beside *each* item below, indicate the degree of the problem by a check mark (✓)	0 Not at all	1 Just a little	2 Pretty much	3 Very much
1. Picks at things (nails, fingers, hair, clothing).				
2. Sassy to grown-ups.				
3. Problems with making or keeping friends.				
4. Excitable, impulsive.				
5. Wants to run things.				
6. Sucks or chews (thumb; clothing; blankets).				
7. Cries easily or often.				
8. Carries a chip on his shoulder.				
9. Daydreams.				
10. Difficulty in learning.				
11. Restless in the "squirmy" sense.				
12. Fearful (of new situations; new people or places; going to school).				
13. Restless, always up and on the go.				
14. Destructive.				
15. Tells lies or stories that aren't true.				
16. Shy.				
17. Gets into more trouble than others same age.				
18. Speaks differently from others same age (baby talk; stuttering; hard to understand).				
19. Denies mistakes or blames others.				
20. Quarrelsome.				
21. Pouts and sulks.				
22. Steals.				
23. Disobedient or obeys but resentfully.				

Based on a 1975 questionnaire developed by C. Keith Conners, Ph.D. and distributed by Abbott Laboratories. Used by permission.

QUESTIONNAIRE (CONT)

	0	1	2	3
24. Worries more than others (about being alone; illness or death).				
25. Fails to finish things.				
26. Feelings easily hurt.				
27. Bullies others.				
28. Unable to stop a repetitive activity.				
29. Cruel.				
30. Childish or immature (wants help he shouldn't need; clings; needs constant reassurance).				
31. Distractibility or attention span a problem.				
32. Headaches.				
33. Mood changes quickly and drastically.				
34. Doesn't like or doesn't follow rules or restrictions.				
35. Fights constantly.				
36. Doesn't get along well with brothers or sisters.				
37. Easily frustrated in efforts.				
38. Disturbs other children.				
39. Basically an unhappy child.				
40. Problems with eating (poor appetite; up between bites).				
41. Stomachaches.				
42. Problems with sleep (can't fall asleep; up too early; up in the night).				
43. Other aches and pains.				
44. Vomiting or nausea.				
45. Feels cheated in family circle.				
46. Boasts and brags.				
47. Lets self be pushed around.				
48. Bowel problems (frequently loose; irregular habits; constipation).				

Merely add the scores from the following questions: 4, 10, 11, 13, 19, 25, 30, 31, 33, and 37. The other answers don't count. The highest possible score is 30. The lowest is 0. Record the type and amount of activity-modifying drugs your child is on at the time you do the scoring. If you write lightly in pencil, you can erase your answers and repeatedly check your child's progress in the future.

In general, most truly hyperactive children have scores over 17. The higher the score or nearer the score is to 30, the more hyperactive your child is. When scores are above 17, parents are distraught. If scores are above 25, parents are desperate. Parents continue to appear to need more help for their child until the scores are below 8. Some children have low scores, but are problems because of their behavior, rather than activity. This type of test may not give a valid indication of isolated behavior-type problems. For example, the diet in chapter 4 may cause your child to improve to a remarkable degree, but the score might not change if the major problems are irritability, frequent crying, and angry behavior.

The Hyperkinesis Parent's Questionnaire is available only to physicians to help them follow the progress of a child on a treatment program. No norms have been established, so the scores cannot be used for diagnostic purposes.

THE VITAMIN CONTROVERSY

How important is nutrition in relation to hyperactivity?

We simply do not know to what extent optimum nutrition will help hyperactive children, because this has not been studied adequately. There is agreement that we all need vitamins, minerals, complete proteins, carbohydrates, essential fatty acids, enzymes and trace metals or elements for proper health and to prevent disease. Many medical physicians and some nutrition advisers believe a balanced diet will supply these essential needs for both children and adults. Feeding a high quality diet to a hyperactive child, however, cannot be equated to high quality nutrition. Complex factors in digestion, absorption, and transportation within the body may be faulty. Optimum nutrition depends upon a number of factors, and all must function well from the time the food enters the mouth until the nutrients reach the body cells. If one cog in the machinery is malfunctioning, a deficiency or excess can result. A significant imbalance can cause subtle and eventually overt disease.

A second problem is that our present-day foods are not as nutritious as they previously were because of unnatural methods of farming and modern methods of processing, refining, packaging, and cooking. Our crops are grown in polluted air, watered by polluted water, and sprayed with potentially harmful chemicals and insecticides. Fruits and vegetables grown by present-day methods may appear large and rich in color but often lack not only flavor but essential nutrients.

In addition to the problem of deficiencies in our present food supply, there is the problem that people are not all alike. The physiologic needs of an individual can vary with diet, heredity, age, hormonal influences and daily stresses of normal living. The needs of an individual may be met by an average diet or average supplements, but if one essential nutrient is present in too high or too low an amount in a person's body for a critical period of time, normal cellular function can be altered so that optimum health is not possible. Some families have genetic nutritional weaknesses which create a select need for supplementation. It must be appreciated that subliminal or marginal vitamin deficiencies do not manifest as full-blown diseases but rather as a cluster of vague complaints which signal that a person's health is not ideal. Could the many symptoms so commonly associated with hyperactivity in children be indicative of an early nutritional need? We don't know.

There is some evidence to suggest that vitamins C and E can protect us from the toxic effects of infection and air pollution (Williams and Kalita 1977). Some physicians claim that higher doses of niacin (B_3), calcium pantothenate, pyridoxine (B_6), ascorbic acid (C), and tocopherols (E), plus a diet high in protein but low in carbohydrates (wheat flour), sweets, and salt help hyperactive/learning disabled children (Cott 1977). Lead and copper levels tend to be high, while zinc, potassium and manganese may be low in affected children (von Hilsheimer 1970, 1974).

Until we have more nutrition specialists and knowledge, the public must be as wary of a blanket treatment for all people, which uses "no" or the "usual" amounts of vitamins, as they are of a treatment with massive doses of nutrients.

Nutritional misinformation and faddism are presently stimulating increased interest in research, and in time we should have valid answers. However, until we can determine the exact needs of an individual at a cellular level, we can only measure nutrient levels indirectly by analysis of hair or blood serum (which has a direct interchange with cells), or possibly by analysis of nails.

From these findings both deficiencies and excesses sometimes can be recognized and treated. Careful monitoring at intervals after therapy can indicate when appropriate therapeutic adjustments should be made. If specialist care and monitoring of our nutrition is not realistically possible, then the public must be aware of subtle evidence suggesting deficiency, as well as nutrient toxicity. The requirements needed by an individual patient may lie anywhere between the dose recommended as the minimal daily requirement and a dose known to cause side effects or toxicity in some others. Individualized personal care is the key to optimum body functioning. Our ultimate aim must be to focus upon prevention and health rather than upon drugs and disease.

Which vague general symptoms may indicate early vitamin deficiency?

B_1 (Thiamine)
Loss of appetite, depression, irritability, confusion, loss of memory, inability to concentrate, sensitivity to noise.

B_3 (Niacin)
Anxiety, depression, fatigue, hyperactivity, headache, insomnia, hyperesthesia (increased sensitivity to touch). Later symptoms include: failing vision, hypersensitivity to light and odors, dizziness, dulled sense of taste or salty taste and hallucinations.

B_6 (Pyridoxine)
No specific symptoms. This vitamin is a precursor for at least 50 enzymes necessary for normal body function.

B_{12} (Cyanocobalamine)
Depression, agitation, and hallucinations.

Pantothenic acid
Irritability, depression, tension, numbness, dizziness, and a sullen disposition. This vitamin is needed for stress.

C (Ascorbic acid)
Listlessness and blood vessel problems. Rats need three times as much vitamin C when stressed. Humans apparently also require additional vitamin C for mental and physical stress.

Do vitamins or megavitamins help hyperactive children?

We don't know. Some physicians say they do and others say they do not. Acceptable scientific studies have not been documented which give definitive answers although preliminary research and claims of success suggest this area is worthy of study (Williams 1977). In general, fat-soluble vitamins such as A, D, and K are stored in the liver so they must be taken with caution because an overdose can cause harmful effects. Vitamin E is fat soluble but appears to be nontoxic and free of side effects in doses up to 800 IU. Water-soluble vitamins such as C and B complex seldom cause serious side effects and are claimed by some to be helpful for hyperactive children with learning problems. A water-soluble form of vitamin A is now available. (See also Hoffer 1974, Fredericks 1976, Cheraskin et al. 1974, Newbold 1975, Pfeiffer 1975, Rosenberg and Feldzamen 1974, Stone 1974, Wunderlich 1973.)

Are natural or synthetic vitamins better?

Natural vitamins have ingredients which are lacking in synthetic vitamins. For example, natural vitamin C contains rutin, citrin, and hesperidin which supposedly act as synergists or helpers to increase the therapeutic effects of the vitamin. It is claimed that natural vitamins may be superior because they are a naturally balanced combination of ingredients essential for maximum biologic effect. It is known that synthetic vitamins have the same molecular structure as natural vitamins and in some studies these have been particularly useful when given therapeutically for short-term acute disease or severe deficiency diseases. In short, both seem helpful but the natural appears to have a possible edge in superiority.

What are the known toxic and side effects of some vitamins?

Vitamin A

Toxic effects have been noted in some people using large doses, such as 50,000 IU's per day. These include food craving or loss of appetite, fatigue, bone pain, hair loss, yellow skin, red and swollen gums, tight muscles, joint or muscle aches, headaches and itchy, scaly skin over fingers and palms. A sudden overdose of vitamin A can cause an upset stomach, nausea, vomiting, headache, dizziness, seizures, drowsiness and peeling of the skin.

Vitamin B complex
In general, these can cause side effects, but are *not* considered toxic. In addition, some mold-sensitive patients may react to yeast in B complex vitamins (see appendix B15). Below are common side effects of the individual B-type vitamins. If these symptoms appear during drug use, lower the dose and discuss the effects with your physician.

Vitamin B_1 (Thiamine HCL)
This can cause nausea, restlessness, sweating, fast heartbeat, swelling, or edema of tissues (sudden weight gain), trembling, low blood pressure, liver palm (redness on lower half of palm with a pale area in the center.

Vitamin B_2 (Riboflavin)
This can cause itching and tingling of the extremities.

Vitamin B_3 (Niacin or Niacinamide [Nicotinamide] or Nicotinic Acid)
Niacin and niacinamide can be used interchangeably. If one causes an undesirable side effect, the other or a lower dose of both may be tried. Niacin commonly causes warm or flushed skin, especially in fair or redhaired persons. This harmless effect often stops during the first weeks of treatment. Niacinamide occasionally causes nausea. Sometimes in adults, it causes depression or brown skin pigmentation. Nicotinic acid may cause heartburn, and occasionally, depression.

Vitamin B_6 (Pyridoxine)
Overdose is unlikely. Diarrhea or nausea is sometimes noted if the dosage is excessive.

Vitamin B_{12}
No problems with safety.

Vitamin B_{15} (Pangamic Acid)
This is presently being evaluated for safety and effectiveness.

Vitamin B Biotin
Doses as high as 0.9 to 1.8 mg are considered safe.

Vitamin B Choline
Overdose is highly unlikely.

Vitamin B Folic Acid
Overdose is unlikely. Folic acid can damage the nervous system if it is taken without vitamin B_{12} to treat pernicious anemia.

Vitamin B Inositol
Overdose is unlikely.

Vitamin B-PABA (Para-aminobenzoic Acid)
Apparently safe.
Pantothenic Acid or Calcium Pantothenate
Apparently safe.

Vitamin C
Rarely this can cause diarrhea, gas, activation of a preexisting peptic ulcer, or a need to urinate more often than usual.

Vitamin D
A toxic dose can be as little as 2,000 or as much as 15,000 IU's per day. The dose needed by one child may be toxic to another. Symptoms include nausea, vomiting, diarrhea, weight loss, thirst, joint pain, and excessive urination (especially at night). Prolonged excessive use can cause kidney damage, hardening of the blood vessels, and elevation of the blood pressure due to calcium deposits in the tissues.

Vitamin E
Toxicity related to this vitamin has been debated. A dose of 800 IU's per day is considered nontoxic. Larger doses for prolonged periods can questionably cause muscle weakness, gastrointestinal upset, elevated blood pressure, and, possibly, reproductive dysfunction.

Vitamin K
This can cause vomiting or blood clotting problems.

Most undesirable effects from vitamins disappear when the dosage is lowered or the vitamin is no longer used.

How can you check the dose of vitamin C you are taking?

Purchase one ounce of 10 percent silver nitrate from your druggist. Mix equal parts of urine with the nitrate solution; for example, twenty drops of each. If the color of the urine changes to white, the vitamin C level is low. If the color is gray, it means the blood has enough vitamin C and a little is spilling into the urine. If the color becomes black, it means vitamin C is being excreted in your urine because the body has more than it can use. These are only rough measures, but they may help you to keep the level in the gray or moderate range.

Be careful when you handle silver nitrate that you don't spill it.

It turns almost everything it touches, including your fingertips, black. Glass is not affected.

What clue might indicate a vitamin B₆ or pyridoxine deficiency?

A craving for highly seasoned or salted foods may indicate a lack of vitamin B_6. This deficiency causes a loss of taste, so foods need more seasoning to give them flavor. The patient may use ketchup on everything. Vegetables are often refused. Patients who are B_6 deficient are said to be unable to recall dreams.

Will trace metals or minerals help hyperactive children?

We don't know. Some physicians claim that the total care of a hyperactive child should include evaluation of the patient's copper, zinc, lead, iron, mercury, magnesium, sodium, potassium, calcium, manganese, cobalt, chromium, and iodine levels. Until more scientific research is carried out, no one will have the answer for certain. An excess or deficiency of any of these can surely cause the body to function improperly. Don't try to treat your child. Check with your physician. He can do tests to determine if your child's blood levels of these metals or minerals are correct. Hair analyses can be informative, but may be deceptive, because many shampoos contain trace metals (Pfeiffer 1975, Schroeder 1973).

Is there any way you can spot a zinc deficiency?

Look at your child's fingernails. Zinc deficiency can cause little white flecks or specks on nails that may be dull or more brittle than normal. Stretch marks similar to those seen in women who have had babies, may be noted on the back, arms, or legs. The child's hair may be brittle and lack color. Some may complain of cold extremities and poor circulation, feeling faint, arthritis, or joint aches. An unusual sensitivity to light might be present, causing sunglasses to be worn when it is not sunny. Another clue to a possible zinc deficiency is a lack of sensitivity to pain.

Some physicians claim that by correcting, in particular, low zinc and high copper levels, hyperactivity can be reduced in some children. A high copper level often can be reduced merely by raising the zinc level to normal. This effect may be enhanced if manganese and pyridoxine are also supplied.

Is there a clue for a magnesium deficiency?

Persons with this type of deficiency often dislike green vegetables, which contain magnesium. Patients also may be overly sensitive to noise, loud sounds, and music.

Any special tips concerning vitamins and minerals?

Yes. Don't buy them if they contain corn, sugar, or artificial colors or flavors, if these are a problem for your child.

Three acceptable sources are:

WILLNER CHEMISTS
   330 Lexington Avenue
   New York, NY 10016
   (212) 685-2538
VITAL LIFE
   P.O. Box 618
   Carlsbad, CA 92008
   (714) 729-3919
BRONSON PHARMACEUTICALS
   4526 Rinetti Lane
   LaCanada, CA 91011
   (213) 790-2646

Check at health food stores for other brands, such as Carlson, Solgar, etc.

What range of megavitamins or minerals do some physicians suggest?

There are variations but, in general, doses are started at low levels and increased if no bad effects are noted. Children who respond are usually better within two to six months (Williams and Kalita 1977, Newbold 1975).

RANGE OF VITAMINS AND MINERALS

	Under 35 pounds	Over 45 pounds
Vitamin B₁ (Thiamine)	50 to 100 mg.* a day	100 to 1,000 mg. a day
Vitamin C	500 to 1,000 mg. a day	1,000 to 3,000 mg. a day
Vitamin B₃ (Niacin, Niacinamide, or Nicotinic Acid)	500 to 1,000 mg. a day	1,000 to 3,000 mg. a day
Vitamin B₆ (Pyridoxine)	100 to 200 mg. a day	200 to 400 mg. a day
Calcium Pantothenate	200 to 300 mg. a day	400 to 600 mg. a day
Vitamin E (mixed tocopherols)	50 to 100 mg. a day	1500 mg. a day
Manganese	Children who appear to respond to vitamin B₆ and zinc sometimes improve to a greater degree if manganese is also given in a dose of 3 to 5 mg. The chelated form is more easily digested.	
Zinc	10 to 15 mg. a day	
Magnesium	100 to 350 mg. a day	
Calcium	250 to 750 mg. a day	
Lecithin granules	8 to 15 mg. a day	

*1,000 mg. = 1 gm.

The above should not be tried without supervision and advice from your physician. There are many complexities and high doses of one vitamin or mineral may lower another to a level which might cause difficulty. Don't be your own physician. This information is given to make you more knowledgeable about what is being prescribed and why, not as home therapy. Delay in treating a medical symptom can be dangerous. For this reason, don't try to treat your child's symptoms with vitamins. Check with your physician.

THE SUGAR CONTROVERSY

Is hypoglycemia related to hyperactivity or fatigue?

Hypoglycemia, or low blood sugar, can cause underachievement in school, hostility, and unacceptable behavior, but not overactivity. It commonly causes nervous fatigue, exhaustion, depression, confusion, anxiety, dizziness, headaches, muscle aches, trouble sleeping, excessive sweating, tingling skin, cold hands and feet, and midmorning or late afternoon light-headedness. Affected persons are sleepy and tired after a longer-than-normal night's sleep. A craving for sweets and sugar exists and can lead to obesity. Our brains need sugar to function properly and without it, we simply don't feel well. Our body cells need sugar for energy.

Some physicians have noted that some hyperactive children appear to have abnormalities in their metabolism of glucose, but solid scientific documentation is not presently available (Weiss and Kaufman 1971, Buckley 1972, Williams and Kalita 1977).

What causes hypoglycemia?

In some people we do not know what causes it. Low blood sugar can be caused by eating too much or too little sugar. Let me explain. Normally, there is a delicate balance in your body. The supply meets the demand. If your blood sugar or glucose becomes too high, insulin is released and it lowers the sugar level, causing the excess to be stored in your liver in the form of glycogen. If your blood-sugar level becomes too low, glucagon and other enzymes or hormones are released which cause the liver to give up the stored sugar or glycogen, so the blood-sugar level rises. In most persons the delicate balance works with amazing precision and no problems arise. This balance, however, can be upset by problems related to:

A faulty pancreas causing faulty insulin production
Liver damage or liver enzyme deficiency
Insufficient hormones from the adrenal or pituitary glands
The ingestion of certain drugs or toxins
Malabsorption of sugar from the intestines
Kidney malfunction causing a loss of sugar in the urine

There is a splinter group of physicians who are investigating to determine if food or chemical sensitivities could cause the pancreas to become hyperactive. Much more time and study is needed to evaluate scientifically this possible relationship. It has been suggested that an inordinate number of hyperactive children react in an unusual manner to sugar and have a flat glucose-tolerance curve, but no solid documentation is available at this time (Cott 1977, Williams and Kaufman 1977).

In simple, specific terms, what can go wrong when you have hypoglycemia?

Too much sugar eaten
If you always eat too much sugar, your pancreas gets into high

gear and overproduces insulin, which in turn causes too much blood sugar to be stored in the liver. There is not enough left in the blood. This is called functional hypoglycemia and is a common form of this problem. If this is the cause of your problem, you must stop eating so much sugar. Your pancreas may stop overshooting its mark. When you feel symptoms associated with low blood sugar beginning, don't eat sugar, eat protein; for example, meat, cheese, or eggs. These protein foods will provide slowly released glucose, which your pancreas can handle properly. You will feel much better than if you ate sugar. On a regular basis, try to eat less cake, cookies, and starchy foods and drink less coffee, tea, cola, and alcohol.

Too little sugar released into the blood

Liver Disease. Your problem can be in your liver. If the enzymes or hormones which release glycogen (sugar) from the liver don't function properly, you may have low blood sugar, even though the liver warehouse is storing a bountiful sugar supply. In other patients, the liver is damaged and unable to store sugar.

Pituitary or Adrenal Insufficiency. These glands normally produce substances which can directly or indirectly raise the blood sugar. If the glands don't function properly, low blood sugar can result.

Malabsorption. Some intestinal problems interfere with absorption so the foods you eat which contain sugar are unable to provide sugar for your blood.

Alcoholism. Alcohol cannot be substituted for food. Like sugar, it is metabolized quickly in the body. Alcohol provides very temporary help for low blood sugar. If you drink and don't eat sugar or foods to supply glucose, there is an inadequate liver reserve to help if your blood sugar level falls.

Caffeine (Coffee, Tea, Cola) and Tobacco. These items stimulate the adrenal glands to release adrenaline, which raises the blood-sugar level. A relative excess of insulin is released, which can lower the blood sugar too much, causing hypoglycemia.

Too much sugar being stored

Tumors of the pancreas (which are very rare) can produce too much insulin, which lowers the blood sugar too much. The pancreas oversupplies and hypoglycemia results. A diabetic does the same thing when he takes an overdose of insulin.

What is a glucose tolerance test?

This is a test to see if your blood-sugar and insulin levels are properly balanced. Will a high blood-sugar level cause just enough insulin to be released to lower your blood sugar to a normal level? This test tells you the answer. A blood sample is taken at the beginning of the test to see what your blood-sugar level is at that time. You are then given a calculated amount of sugar solution to drink, depending upon your weight. At different intervals of time, for about five or six hours, samples of blood are taken to see what happens to your blood-sugar level.

Blood-sugar levels are recorded in milligrams percent (mg%). Normally, the level is about 80 or 90 mg% at the start of the test because you are requested to eat nothing for twelve hours beforehand. The blood level normally rises during the first hour of the test to about 130 to 220 mg%. During the final three hours of the test, the blood sugar gradually falls to the level it was at the start of the test. If the blood-sugar level rises higher than normal and stays high for several hours, your pancreas may not be producing insulin properly. You may have diabetes and need to take insulin. If your blood sugar rises just a little and then falls 20 mg% below the original blood level, or from 80 to 60 mg%, something is wrong. Your blood level at the end of the test may be normal, but if the blood level dipped too low during the test, it may indicate a problem. This is commonly seen with what is called functional hypoglycemia (see above). Sometimes the glucose blood level stays about the same throughout a glucose-tolerance test. This flat-type curve also may indicate hypoglycemia.

Which rules help with glucose-tolerance-test interpretation?

Interpreting glucose-tolerance curves is not always uniform by all physicians, but the following may be helpful (Newbold 1975):

· After drinking the sugar solution, your previous blood level should double. For example, if the initial level was 80 mg%, it should rise to about 160 mg%.
· The blood-sugar level should not fall at any point during the test below 60 mg% or more than 20 mg% below the fasting level.
· During the test, there should not be a greater than 50 mg% drop during any single hour period. For example, a fall from 140 mg% to 75 mg% in one hour is too much.

· If you perspire, become dizzy, weak, confused, depressed, nauseated, or develop a headache or feel your heart beating fast, ask for an *immediate* blood-sugar determination. If this happens, it means that your blood sugar may be too low at that particular time. Fifteen minutes later, your blood level may no longer be low and the correct diagnosis may be missed.

THE LIGHT AND RADIATION CONTROVERSY

Dr. John Ott of Sarasota, Florida has written a book (1976) explaining many fascinating observations in relation to the effect of different wavelengths of light on plants, animals, and humans. In one study with Dr. Lewis Mayron and others of Chicago (1974), he showed that full-spectrum light with radiation shields decreased hyperactivity in children in two classrooms when compared to two other rooms in which standard cool-white fluorescent light was used. The cool-white light lacks wavelengths of light which they believe to be essential for normal activity in some children. They stress that all fluorescent lights need radiation shielding.

3 · Questions Most People Ask about Allergy

This chapter tells you how you can determine if allergies are present in your family by talking to or looking at your relatives. It explains common causes of allergies and how you can effectively eliminate many of these. It details, in particular, how to try to determine which foods might be causing an allergy.

Lots of people know they have allergies, but many others don't realize that allergies are their problem (Rapp 1972a, 1974). They think coughs are due to cigarettes, their stuffy noses are sinus troubles, and their headaches are from their bosses. Fill in the form on the following pages carefully. Does it apply to anyone in your family—your children, parents, sisters, or brothers? You may find that some relatives fit into one category, while others do not. Remember, everything listed on the form can be due to medical problems entirely unrelated to allergy. If you have many relatives who have typical allergy symptoms, it is certainly possible that allergy may be the cause of some of your child's or your family's atypical or unusual medical problems. The atypical problems include hyperactivity as well as many other allergic-tension-fatigue syndrome symptoms (see chapter 1).

Even if your child's activity problems are not related to allergy, the questions and answers in this chapter may help you, if you or any other member of your family has allergies.

What makes a face look allergic?

Look for black, blue or red circles under the eyes. These tend to appear after a person gets near or eats something to which he is allergic. Another clue is bags under the eyes. Some children have puffiness directly below the eyes and others also have little bags below the outer edge of each eye. Deep creases or wrinkles under

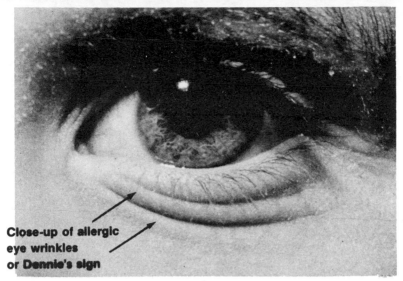

Close-up of allergic eye wrinkles or Dennie's sign

Photographs by Robert Mathibe (Buffalo, New York)

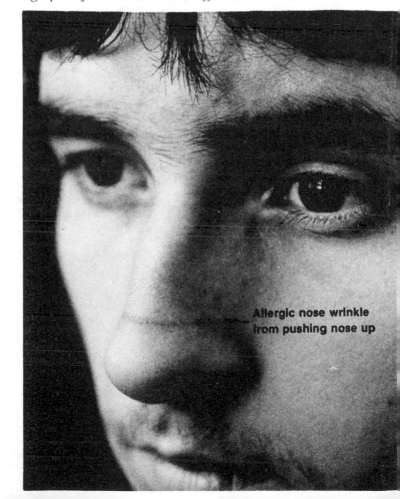

Allergic nose wrinkle from pushing nose up

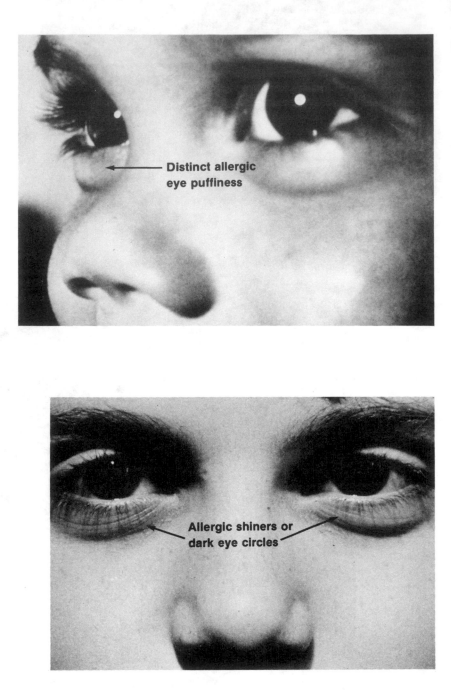

Distinct allergic eye puffiness

Allergic shiners or dark eye circles

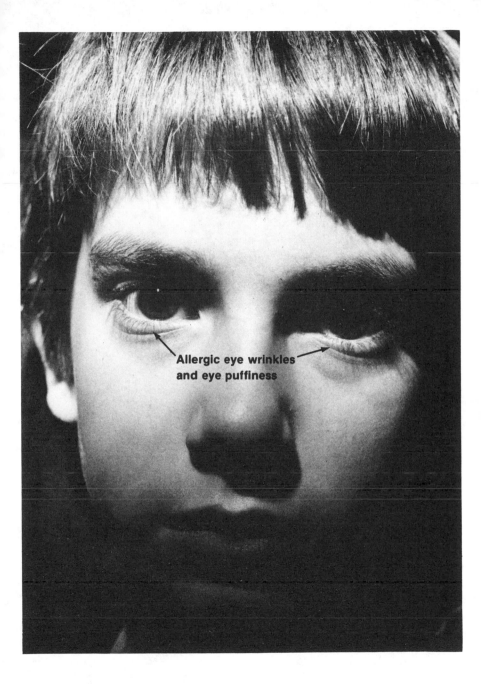

Allergic eye wrinkles and eye puffiness

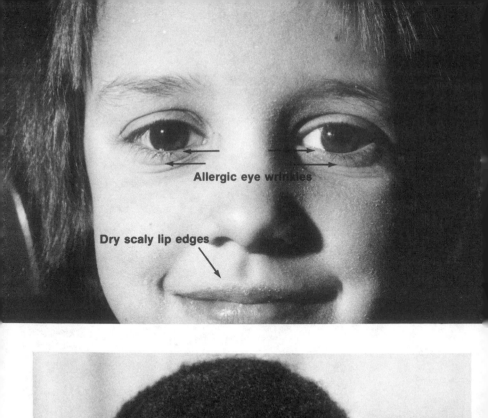

Allergic eye wrinkles

Dry scaly lip edges

Allergic eye
puffiness or
bags under
eyes

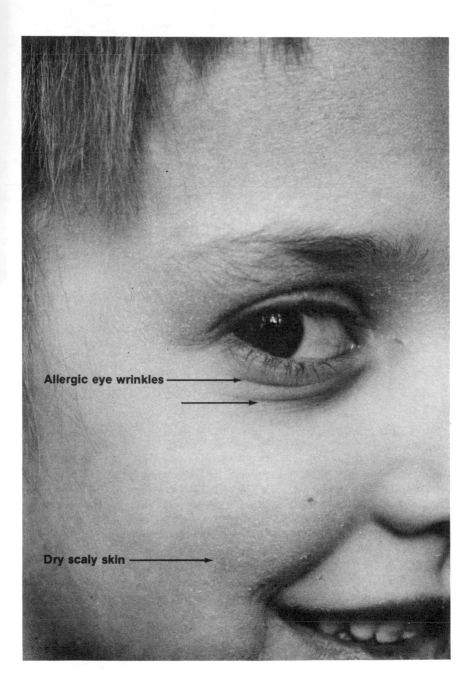

Allergic eye wrinkles

Dry scaly skin

the eyes are typical of persons with allergy. Many have only one wrinkle, but persons with eczema, in particular, may have several.

Push the tip of your nose upward. This causes a crease which will disappear if you don't rub your nose often. People who rub their nose this way frequently cause the crease to remain all the time. Children with nose allergy sometimes wiggle their nose like a bunny rabbit. They can't breathe through their nose so they tend to breathe with their mouth gaping open. This can sometimes cause dental problems and a need for orthodontia.

Some persons with food problems tend to have a rash around their mouth or cracked dry lips. The borders or margins of the lips may look swollen or puffy. Cracks or irritation may be noted in the corners of their mouths. Children with food, toothpaste, or bubblegum problems often lick their lips in excess, all year round, not only during the winter months. In others, lip-licking may be merely a nervous habit.

Some children develop red, rougelike patches on their cheeks or red ears or dark eye circles after eating a food that causes allergy (Marks 1977).

POSSIBLE COMMON SYMPTOMS OF ALLERGY

Nose Allergy   Yes/No

Nose symptoms? _____
   warm months?_____
   cold months? _____
   all year? _____
Stuffy nose? _____
Watery runny nose? _____
Sneeze several times in a
     row? _____
Rub nose upwards?_____
Wiggle nose? _____
Pick nose? _____
Clear throat often? _____
One cold after another,
    but not sick?_____
   how often per month?_____
   other times? _____
Nosebleeds? _____
   how often? _____

Chest Allergy   Yes/No

Wheeze or asthma?_____
   with infection?_____
   other times? _____
Cough or wheeze? _____
   with laughter? _____
   with exercise? _____
   with cold air? _____
   with cold drinks?_____
   at night? _____
   when it's damp outside?_____

Skin Allergy   Yes/No

Eczema or atopic dermatitis? _____
Itchy rash in arm or leg creases? ___
Cracked toes or fingernails? _____
Hives or welts? _____
Itchy skin—no rash? _____
Itchy rash on body? _____

Eye Allergy   Yes/No

Puffy eyes? _____

Wrinkles under eyes? _____

Black circles under eyes? _____

Itchy eyes? _____

Red eyes? _____

Watery eyes? _____

Both eyes affected? _____

Burning eyes? _____

Painful eyes? _____

Eyes light sensitive? _____

POSSIBLE ATYPICAL SYMPTOMS OF ALLERGY

Ear Allergy   Yes/No

Recurrent fluid behind
  eardrums? _____

On and off hearing
  trouble? _____

Ear popping? _____

Flushed, red ear lobes? _____

Ringing in ears? _____

Dizziness? _____

Urinary Problems:
Bladder or Kidney   Yes/No

Wet pants in daytime? _____

Wet bed at night? _____

  how many times
    per week? _____

  how many times
    per month? _____

Recurrent bladder
  infections? _____

Other kidney or bladder
  problems? _____

Need to urinate at night? _____

Pain with urination? _____

Frequent need to urinate
  during the day? _____

Blood in urine? _____

Burn when passing urine? _____

Need to rush to urinate? _____

Do urine problems
  recur at specific times
  each year? _____

Intestinal Allergy   Yes/No

Colic over age 6 months
  when infant? _____

Unable to drink milk as
  infant? _____

Swelling of face or lips? _____

Soreness of edges of lips? _____

Irritation of corners of
  mouth? _____

Excess drooling? _____

Mottled "bald" patches
  on tongue? _____

Deep grooves or fissures
  in tongue? _____

Excessive throat mucus? _____

Itchy roof of mouth? _____

Canker sores? (ulcers on
  gums, inside cheeks) _____

Bad breath? _____

Clucking throat sounds? _____

Frequent bellyaches? _____

Frequent nausea? _____

Excess belly gas? _____

Bloated belly? _____

Diarrhea—often? _____

Constipation—often? _____

Itchy rectal area? _____

Ulcers, gastric or peptic? _____

Colitis? _____

Miscellaneous	Yes/No
Headache?	
Growing pains?	
Muscle aches?	
Pain in neck or shoulder?	
Backaches?	
Leg cramps?	
Joint aches?	
Tingling in arms and legs?	
Excessive perspiration?	
Oversensitive to cold?	
Excessive infections?	
Frequent fevers without infections?	
Vaginal itching or irritation?	
Irregular heartbeat?	
Sudden rapid heartbeat	

Skin Allergy	Yes/No
Easy bruising?	
Tender sore skin spots?	
Swollen face or feet?	
Puffy fingers or hands?	

Nervous System	Yes/No
Constant wiggling about?	
Irritable?	
Hyperactive? Restless?	
Clumsy?	
Listless? Tired?	
Hostile? Fights a lot?	
Cries often or easily?	
Unhappy?	
Behavior problem?	
Seems "spaced-out"?	
Talks nonsense?	
Talks too much?	
Sleeps poorly?	
Nightmares?	
Sleepy and tired in A.M.?	
Sleepy after eating?	
Sleepy after napping?	
Unexplained depression?	
Seizures?	
Stutters?	
Good vocabulary but can't read?	
Can't draw, print, or write?	
Can't concentrate or poor attention span?	
Dislikes loud noise?	
Dislikes bright lights?	
Dislikes many odors?	

What causes allergies?

There are many types of allergy, but the most common ones are caused by one or more of the following:

Things inside your home. You may have to change your home.
Things outside your home. You may need allergy tests for pollens and mold spores and, possibly, allergy-injection therapy.
Things which you eat. You may have to change your diet.

Are different allergies caused by different things?

Yes, but in general, whether your problem is your nose, lungs, skin, brain, or elsewhere, the treatment is often the same. Change your house or your diet or get treatment for pollens and molds (or possibly dust and other things known to cause allergy). Some people don't follow advice unless they pay for personal attention. If you'd prefer personal attention, see an allergist. If you want to try to help yourself, remember, if you do half of what is suggested, you may notice 50 percent improvement.

How can you tell which things might be causing symptoms and help yourself or your family?

Regardless of age, and regardless of which part of the body is affected by allergy, the approach is similar and systematic.

· *Is it something in your house?* The clues which give you the answer: Are you or your family, always or sometimes, free of symptoms when away from home, that is, when visiting, vacationing, camping, or in a hospital, and worse as soon as you return? Are you worse in the colder months when you are inside more often? Are you worse in the morning or in certain rooms in your home? Have you noticed that dust, feathers, pets, a moldy basement, or home odors seem to bother you? If your answer is yes, part or all of your problem may be due to your home (see appendix E1 which details exactly what you can do to help yourself). If making your home, particularly the bedroom, more allergy-free does not help your winter symptoms, you may have to be skin-tested for certain home items that often cause allergy. These include dust, feathers, kapok, pets, mold spores, certain odors, and chemicals. By avoidance or treatment with allergy-extract medicine, your symptoms may be relieved. Chemical sensitivities, that is, gas fumes, oil, plastic, perfume, and so on, may present a difficult, almost impossible, challenge (see appendix E3).

· *Is the problem due to something in the outside air?* To answer this, consult the "Pollen Calendar," Appendix D. Do the symptoms that bother your child or family recur or seem particularly severe only during certain warm months each year when specific pollens or mold spores are in the air? If every year the symptoms recur, almost on the same day, and magically disappear or diminish a few weeks later, this may be the answer. Do your symptoms seem worse when the air is heavily polluted? Contaminated air can cause particular difficulty on windy or foggy days. Insect, garden, and lawn sprays or fertilizers may be particularly offensive.

Can hyperactivity be related to exposure within schools?

Many exposures in school are capable of causing symptoms in children (Blume 1968). Hyperactivity, fatigue, behavior and personality problems, headaches, and abdominal complaints are common, as well as traditional allergies such as asthma, a stuffy or runny nose, itchy watery eyes, or hives. Parents should be cautious not to attribute all school-associated symptoms to an emotional problem or dislike of school (Buisseret 1978). Be suspicious of something in school if your child's problems are noted only on school days, not on weekends, vacations, or holidays.

If your child seems well when he leaves home but is ill by the time he returns, the cause may be some school exposure. If symptoms routinely occur between 1:00 and 2:00 P.M., think of the school lunch. If only certain days or times are repeatedly involved, think of classes or contacts just prior to the onset of symptoms. Some children routinely become ill after gym or art class, in particular. If symptoms are sudden or strange, ask your child what happened in school that was unusual on that particular day. A teacher may be able to help pinpoint the cause of your child's symptoms once it is known that foods, odors, and contacts can have adverse and, at times, surprising effects in some children (and adults). Alert the teacher to the dark eye circles, the glassy look in the eyes, the red ear lobes, or red cheek spots which so often help a mother recognize the onset of an allergic reaction.

Potential School Sources of Difficulty

School Lunch. Food coloring, sugar, chocolate, tomato, peanut butter, grapes, wheat, eggs, dairy products, citrus, apple, corn products, carbonated beverages, or foods with preservatives or additives. Symptoms usually occur within an hour after eating but delayed reactions may not be noticed for several hours.

Classroom. Chalk dust, chemically treated mimeo or copy paper, correction fluid, plastic schoolbags or pencil holders, plastic or fiberglass drapes, synthetic or chemically treated wool carpets, rubber carpet padding, moldy plants, tobacco odors, partial-spectrum fluorescent light, fur- or feather-covered pets, their excrement or feed, and any cosmetics worn by students or teachers.

Art Class.   Magic marker pens, rubber or spray cements, glue, paste, glaze, tempera, water or oil paint, paint thinners or solvents, India or linoleum ink, clay, odor of kilns for pottery, all types of aerosols, dried plants, flowers, or leaves (molds).

Woodwork or Metal Shop.   Odor of paint, paint thinners, lacquers, shellac, plastic, smoke, burning items, or sawdust.

Chemistry.   Odor or any chemical or gas emitted from an experiment, odor of Bunsen burner or gas fumes.

Printing Class.   Odor of ink or cleaning solutions, ditto or copy paper, stencil or mimeograph paper.

Gym Class.   Dust or mold in gym, locker rooms, or in tumbling mats, odor of chlorine, fungicides or molds in pool area, pollen, lawn, or air pollutants when taking gym outside school.

Lavatories or Showers.   Odor of Lysol or pine-scented cleaning solutions, deodorizers, germicides, hairspray, perfume, after-shave lotions, fingernail polish or remover, depilatories, hand lotion, scented body powders, underarm deodorants, and tobacco.

Cooking Class.   Odor of egg, peanut, other nuts, fish, or boiled potato. Contact with sifted flour. Odor of gas stove or hot grease, especially if exhaust fan does not function properly.

Cleaning.   Any janitorial item such as soap, aerosol cleaner, dusting compound, floor wax, furniture, woodwork or metal polish.

Heating.   The odor of raw or burning gas, oil, or coal, or their fumes when improperly vented. Dust in ductwork or molds in humidifiers or air conditioners.

Maintenance.   Fresh paint, new floor covering, pesticide, insecticide, or exterminator chemicals, odors from lawn equipment, lawn fertilizers, and asphalt repair products.

Miscellaneous.   Special projects associated with school plays, bazaars, or holidays. The preparation of Christmas presents for parents in particular seems to be associated with contact of sensitizing substances.

School Bus.   Odor of exhaust or gasoline fumes, plastic, rubber, or bus upholstery, perfume, hairspray, or tobacco.

If your child is well when he leaves home and ill by the time he arrives at school, consider not only the school bus, but also what was eaten for breakfast. If the weekday breakfast differs from that eaten on weekends, a food might be at fault.

How are pollen and mold problems treated?

First, you can try to make your home more "allergy-free" at the time of year when you are bothered (see appendix E1). If your home is moldy, try the suggestions in appendix E2. You can tell if your house is moldy if the shower area looks moldy or smells musty; if the basement is or has been flooded and smells damp or if you use a room vaporizer so often the bedroom has a moldy smell. Molds often grow in paste under wallpaper or along rubber fittings in a refrigerator. They can also grow in humidifiers and air conditioners.

There are room air purifiers which remove pollens and molds from the air. These not only appear to help if used during the pollen season, but may relieve winter symptoms due to dust, feathers, pets, and so on. The odor of HEPA or ozone filters can aggravate some allergic patients.

Following the above suggestions often helps, but may not completely relieve a patient's symptoms. Many people need to see an allergist to be skin-tested for pollens and molds so an allergy-extract medicine can be prepared. Injection therapy for molds or pollens often partially or totally relieves seasonal symptoms. Always remember, however, that the treatment should not be worse than the disease. If the seasonal symptoms are mild, require little medicine, and do not interfere with normal activities, no special treatment may be needed until more difficulty is en-countered.

There are, however, some studies that indicate that at least 30 to 50 percent of the children who have hay fever, subsequently wheeze (Johnstone 1957). For this reason, some allergists advocate treatment of hay fever so that the problem will not progress to asthma. A warning that a hay-fever patient may be developing chest allergies is that he or she experiences prolonged coughing, especially with exercise, laughter, or emotional upsets, during the pollen season. If you notice this, be sure to check with your doctor.

Many persons with warm-weather problems forget that seasonal foods may cause symptoms during the summer months. Fresh fruits, corn, melon, tomatoes and summer-type citrus fruit or dyed beverages may cause seasonal symptoms. Bananas and melons, for example, may cause symptoms only during the ragweed pollen season (see Appendix D).

Because most people are outside more during the summer months, air pollution of various types often causes symptoms.

How can you tell if your child's or family's health problem may be due to a food?

If you answer "yes" to many of the following, food may be a cause of the problem.

· Did an allergy symptom appear during the first year of life? Regardless of a person's present age, if the problem started in infancy, think of foods first.

· Was excessive mucus a problem during infancy, or is it a problem now?

· Was the infant formula changed often, without helping?

· Did colic last longer than three to six months (Frazier 1974)?

· As a baby, was irritability and inability to sleep a problem (Crook 1973, 1977, 1978)?

· Was milk a problem during the child's infant period, although, later on, it seemed to be all right. If this was noted, milk again may be a problem. For example, milk might cause colic or eczema during infancy, a stuffy, runny, watery nose from the age of two to five years and then cause asthma or hyperactivity (Dickey 1976a). The same food can affect different areas of the body, at different times in a person's life (see the case history of M. L. in chapter 1).

· Do you have relatives with known food allergies? Which foods? Specific food problems tend to be found in families, especially milk (Gerrard 1973, Breneman 1978; see appendix B5). If one food caused one child to have a symptom, maybe that same food is causing another symptom in another child or a parent (Tuft 1973).

· Are some foods craved more than others? These may be the ones! The food a person would miss most is often the most likely to cause symptoms. Coffee, chocolate, sweets, colored pop, wheat (bread, cakes, cookies), alcohol.

· Is a food which most people like, intensely disliked? It is unusual for children to dislike milk, ice cream, or chocolate, in particular. An aversion may indicate a food problem. A dislike for squash or liver is understandable, but not for chocolate.

· Does your family have circles under their eyes, puffy eye bags, patchy-appearing tongues, canker sores, sore lips, or lip edges (Speer 1954)? Black eye circles may not be hereditary. They may be the result of a food problem within a family.

· Is anyone's belly unusually bloated? Is belching, rectal gas, or bad breath a recurrent and frequent problem?

· Does the allergy problem persist in spite of where you travel or visit (Rapp 1974)?

· Are allergy symptoms present every day or intermittently all year long? Are they, possibly, a bit better in the summer or warmer months (Rinkel 1944)?

· Do you feel better when you don't eat? Do you regularly skip meals? Many food allergics feel best if they eat only one large meal in the evening.

· When you have an infection or digestive problem and do not eat, does your nose clear?

· When you fast for a religious celebration or before surgery, do you feel better?

· Do symptoms tend to appear less before you eat and more within an hour or two after eating? Does a particular food repeatedly cause symptoms eight to twelve hours after eating?

· Does the teacher notice your child is often worse after a snack break or lunch? Find out what your child ate that day.

· Do you know some foods which you must avoid because they always cause trouble?

· Do you know some foods which sometimes, repeatedly, seem to cause trouble?

· Have you made your home allergy-free and have you been treated for years with pollen, dust, and other common items found in allergy extracts without satisfactory improvement? In particular, does your nose still run or seem stuffy each day? Is your asthma poorly controlled (Taube 1973)? Do you need daily asthma drugs or cortisone?

· Do you or your family have many typical or unusual symptoms which might indicate allergy (see chapter 3) but because routine allergy skin testing failed to show a cause, you think allergy can't be your problem? Traditional allergy testing is notoriously inaccurate for many foods.

· Does any family member make clucking, snorting, throaty sounds, have a daily postnasal drip or frequent sinus infections or complain about an itchy roof of the mouth, tongue, or lips?

· Do you find you often become drowsy after eating, even when you're well-rested (Miller 1972)?

Can patients have a combined problem?

Sure. Many people with allergies have daily or on-and-off trouble all year, due to things they eat or have in their homes, but are much worse during a pollen season in the warm months. These people have to attack their problems with enthusiasm. They must do *more* before improvement is noted.

If you have a dozen slivers in your finger, it does not help to remove two slivers or put on an ointment. You remove all of them. If five foods are at fault, it may help only a little to detect three of them. If the problem is pollen, dust, molds, pets, and foods, you may not be helped sufficiently if you are treated only for pollens and dust, or only for foods.

Special tips if you think your family has food allergy

· Try the entire family on the diet (appendix B3) for a week or two. Remember, one food can cause problems for several members, but the symptoms may not be the same in all people. Milk, for example, might make one child wet the bed and another hyperactive; it may cause bellyaches in a mother and headaches in a father. It is easier to cook and easier to control the menu if everyone tries the same diet at once. Be sure, however, everyone is in reasonably good health. If there is a question, check with your physician.

· If someone has a daily medical problem think of foods eaten quite often. If it is a rare problem, think of foods eaten infrequently. Although offending foods generally cause symptoms for a few hours, sometimes a problem food can cause symptoms for a full four days after it is eaten.

· If you eat a problem food every day you might not notice that it causes minimal daily difficulty. If you stop eating a food entirely for several weeks before you start to eat it again, even if it is a problem, it may not cause difficulty right away. It may take several days or weeks before the "old" symptoms gradually reappear. Unless this is understood, confusion will persist in the minds of both patients and physicians.

If, however, you eat large amounts of a food on the first day, then avoid that food in any form for five to ten days before eating a normal amount of the food again, you are most apt to see a dramatic reaction to a problem food. Symptoms will often appear within an hour if a food is eaten after the five-to-ten-day strict avoidance diet period (Rinkel and Zeller 1951).

There are exceptions, however. At times, some food reactions consistently recur eight to twelve hours after a food is eaten. Or, sometimes, the food must be eaten for one or more days before symptoms are noted. Eating suspect foods at five-to-ten-day intervals, however, seems to be one of the best ways to increase one's chances of easily and quickly finding valid answers in relation to food problems.

· A number of physicians have found that about ½ to 1 teaspoon of baking soda dissolved in water or fruit juice sometimes helps relieve a food-sensitivity reaction. Many years ago, Dr. Theron Randolph of Chicago recommended a mixture of two-parts baking soda (sodium bicarbonate) and one part potassium bicarbonate (Randolph 1976a). This can be prepared by a pharmacist without a prescription. Some commercial bicarbonate preparations—for example Alka-Seltzer Antacid Formula without Aspirin or citro-carbonate—are available; they are similar to the baking soda-potassium bicarbonate mixture but taste better. Although these help some patients, they do not appear to be as effective as Dr. Randolph's original mixture.

Regardless of the part of the body affected, these alkaline bicarbonate salts may help. While they often relieve hives, itchy skin, bellyaches, or hyperactivity due to dyed food items, they may or may not help nose symptoms or asthma due to food. The preparation can be taken twenty minutes before an offending food is eaten, for example at a birthday party, to prevent an anticipated reaction. If the symptoms have already occurred, bicarbonate may give relief in about twenty minutes, if used immediately.

Although this form of therapy is empirical, scientific double-blind studies are not presently available to document its effectiveness. The theoretical mechanism of action is discussed in detail in a recently written chapter by Dr. Randolph (1976a). Patients who have kidney or heart problems should not use these preparations without their physician's advice.

· If you find milk and dairy products cause symptoms in your family, check with your physician. Growing children need the calcium found in milk. The doctor may prescribe a calcium supplement (see appendix B5).

· Don't try to diet near a holiday or celebration or when traveling or eating in restaurants.

· If you have just placed your family or child on a diet and one member develops an infection, such as a cold, sore throat, or bronchitis, try to stay on the diet. If this proves difficult, merely wait and restart the diet from the beginning later on.

· If you had your child or family on a diet and one person improves, but develops an infection when you are re-adding foods to the diet to find out what happens, you must wait. If you add a food at the same time your child is ill, it will be impossible to tell if infection or the suspect food is causing the difficulty that arises. Stay on the diet until your child is well again and then proceed to add foods back into the diet to find out what happens. If you prefer, stop the diet entirely and start again when the entire family is well.

· If your child is underweight and you are fearful about a diet, first check with your physician. Some children, when deprived of their favorite food, gain weight quickly because that particular food is the major food to which they are sensitive. The appetite can be depressed if a problem food is eaten.

· Diets commonly fail because the patient or family thinks a little mistake won't matter. Some milk-sensitive patients can drink a small amount of milk, but a few are so sensitive that a speck of butter or margarine can cause symptoms for many hours. It is more rewarding for all concerned to do the diet once, and to do it correctly. This may prevent months of dieting without answers, or years of allergies without relief. If you accidentally or deliberately make errors, it may take years before someone can help you figure out the correct answers. A speck of onion in seasoned salt, the little corn or sugar in ketchup, or the dye on or in a pill can cause symptoms in very sensitive patients.

· If you have no medicine at home to treat an allergy and are going to do a diet, you might want to check with your physician. Ryna syrup, Chlor-Trimeton tablets or chewable Novahistine (or Tacaryl) tablets are available to help nose, eye, and skin allergies, such as hives, without a prescription. In most states, Bronkolixir is available to help asthma or an allergic cough. A suggested dosage will be on the bottle.

· Don't forget medicines and vitamins can cause symptoms, too. Flavors, corn, sugar, and dyes in these items cause symptoms in some people. More and more medicines are now available which are dye-corn-sugar-free. Watch and see if certain colors seem to bother your child. If they do, ask your physician for dye-corn-sugar-free medicine or white tablets which can be crushed. Pills that are color-coated can be rinsed with water to remove the dye.

· If you are not sure something can be eaten during a diet trial, don't eat it. Be sure to read through all of Appendix B. Substitutes are listed throughout for foods you may miss. If you don't have time to read labels, don't bother dieting. You must know what you can as well as cannot eat. The lists on these pages will help, but you must double-check every label, reading fully all fine print on front, back, and sides.

· If you repeatedly find a family member is better if a certain food is not eaten and worse if it is eaten, face it. It is hard to accept a sensitivity to a major food such as milk or wheat, but if that is your problem, try not to make excuses.

· Anticipate some problems: For example, if your child can't eat wheat desserts, have some similar tasty substitutes at school for special celebrations. You don't want your child left out if everyone gets a treat. Send items such as potato chips, peanuts, special homemade candy bars or cookies (Dworkin and Dworkin 1974), if you know these don't cause symptoms. Try to use pure food items without additives and chemicals at all times.

The following hints might help:

Breakfast
Meat
Potatoes
Vegetables
Fruit
Coffee Rich (contains dyes) and artificial
sweetener or pure honey or
pure maple syrup on allowed cereal

School Lunch
(Your child can't buy lunch if dieting)
Fruits and Vegetables (fresh or salads)
Homemade soup
Drumstick or pork chop (not breaded)
Ry-Krisp sandwiches (no luncheon meat)
Potato chips (no additives)

Party Time
Read dessert sections of the allergy cookbooks
(see appendix C4)
Soybean-whipped-cream substitute
Soybean milk ice cream (contains sugar)
CaraCoa chocolate bars

If you know, for example, that any food listed above (or any place in this book) cannot be eaten by your child, don't give that to him to eat. He is the exception.

Which method helps detect an intermittent food problem?

Regardless of which symptom your child or you have, if it occurs only once in a while, it may be a food (or odor or contact). If you think it might be a food, the following might prove helpful. Keep a detailed list of what is put into the mouth (foods, beverages, medicines, toothpaste, mouthwash, and so on) for the twelve waking hours before the symptoms began. If you awaken with symptoms, it may be something you ate or touched the afternoon or evening before which is bad for you. If you are fine in the morning, but develop trouble during the day, it may be something you ate, touched, or smelled during that day which is bad. Compare several of these bad-day lists with what you ate, touched, or smelled on days when you were fine all day and the next morning, that is, good days. Cross out everything in both columns. You will be left with only possible food suspects on the bad-day list. Check these one at a time and find out which is at fault. Try eating each suspect food in large amounts every five days. Avoid that food in all forms until each fifth day. If the suspect food is at fault, symptoms often occur within an hour of the time the food is eaten.

Example:

Bad Day	Good Day	Suspect foods
Miller orange juice	Jones grape juice	Miller orange juice
Strawberry Jell-O	Cherry Jell-O	Strawberry (a specific red
~~Beef~~	~~Beef~~	flavor or dye unrelated
~~Potato~~	~~Potato~~	to cherry)

Beef and potatoes are probably not at fault because they caused no difficulty on the good day.

What is a rotary diet?

This special diet is designed so no food is eaten more frequently than every four days. The menu for any day is selected from a list which changes every day for four days; the pattern is repeated over and over again. Initially, no food to which you are sensitive can be eaten more often than once a day (see "Rotary Diet" below).

The purpose of the diet is twofold. First, it helps to detect hidden food offenders. If you remain well until the day you eat a certain food, and repeatedly become ill on the same day in the four-day pattern, it is easy to find the probable culprit food. Once the offending food is omitted from the menu, symptoms on that day of the cycle subside.

The second purpose is to help prevent the development of new food allergies. Physicians knowledgeable about food problems have repeatedly found, for example, that if you place a patient on a milk-free diet and he substitutes orange juice for milk, he often becomes sensitive to orange juice. This tendency can be diminished if the patient repeatedly drinks a different beverage each day for four days.

ROTARY DIET

Each line on the right represents a single food family except those for sweeteners, beverages, soup and miscellaneous items.

	Days 1, 5, 9, etc.
Fruit	Lemon, orange, grapefruit, lime, tangerine, kumquat, citron
	Banana, plantain, arrowroot
	Coconut, date
Vegetables	Carrots, parsnips, celery, parsley
	Sweet potatoes, yams
	Beets, spinach, chard, lamb's quarters (green)
Spices	Celery seed, anise, dill, fennel, cumin, coriander, caraway
	Black and white pepper, peppercorn
	Sea salt
	Nutmeg, mace
Nuts	English walnut, black walnut, pecan, hickory nut, butternut
Meats	All fowl and game birds including chicken, turkey, duck, goose, guinea, pigeon, quail, pheasant, eggs
Sweeteners	Date sugar or beet sugar
Beverages	Tea: Comfrey tea, fennel tea
	Juices may be made and used without added sweeteners from the fruits and

Beverages (cont)	vegetables listed above in any combination desired
Soup	May be made from any of the above ingredients—meat, vegetables, and spices
Miscellaneous	Coconut oil, fats from any bird listed above

Days 2, 6, 10, etc.

Fruit	Grapes, unsulphered raisins—all types (juice pack, water pack, or fresh)
	Strawberries, raspberries, blackberries, dewberries, loganberries, youngberries, boysenberries, rose hips
	Watermelon, cantaloupe, other melons
Vegetables	Cucumber, pumpkin, squash, zucchini
	Peas, black-eyed peas, dry beans, green beans, carob, soybeans, lentils, alfalfa
Spices	Licorice
	Sea salt
Nuts	Cashew, pistachio, mangoes
	Filberts, hazelnuts
	Peanuts
Meats	All pork products—ham, bacon
Seafood	Abalone, snails, squids, clams, mussels, oysters, scallops
	Crab, crayfish, lobster, prawn, shrimp
Sweeteners	CaraCoa, carob syrup, honey
Beverages	Tea: Alfalfa tea, fenugreek
	Juices may be made and used without added sweeteners from the fruits and vegetables listed above in any combination desired
	Soybean milk
Soup	May be made from any of the above ingredients—meat, vegetables, and spices
Miscellaneous	Soybean oil, peanut oil, cottonseed oil
	Pure peanut butter
	Pumpkin, squash, acorn seeds

	Days 3, 7, 11, etc.
Fruit	Apples, pears, quinces
	Mulberries, figs, breadfruit
	Elderberries
	Rhubarb
	Currant, gooseberries
Vegetables	Lettuce, chicory, endive, escarole, artichoke, dandelions
	Potatoes, tomatoes, eggplant, peppers (red and green)
	Onions, asparagus, chives, leeks
Spices	Tarragon
	Chili pepper, paprika, cayenne
	Garlic
	Sea salt
	Basil, savory, sage, oregano, horehound, catnip, spearmint, peppermint, thyme, marjoram, lemon balm
Nuts	Brazil nuts
	Chestnuts
Meats	Lamb, rabbit
Fish	Fresh water: Sturgeon, herring, salmon, whitefish, bass, perch
	Salt water: Sea herring, anchovy, cod, sea bass, sea trout, mackerel, tuna, swordfish, flounder, sole
Sweetener	Saccharin
Beverages	Tea: Kaffir tea, mint tea
	Juices may be made and used without added sweeteners from the fruits and vegetables listed above in any combination desired
Soup	May be made from any of the above ingredients—meat, fish, vegetables, and spices
Miscellaneous	Safflower oil
	Seseme seeds
	Tapioca

Miscellaneous (cont)	Sunflower seeds Olives, green or black Buckwheat
	Days 4, 8, 12, etc.
Fruit	Plums, cherries, peaches, apricots, nectarines, wild cherries Blueberries, huckleberries, cranberries, wintergreen Pawpaw, papaya, papain
Vegetables	Mustard, turnip, radish, horseradish, watercress, cabbage, kraut Chinese cabbage, broccoli, cauliflower, Brussels sprouts, collards Kale, kohlrabi, rutabaga Avocadoes
Spices	Cinnamon, bay leaf Sea salt
Grains	Wheat, corn, rice, oats, barley, rye, wild rice, cane, millet Sorghum, bamboo sprouts
Nuts	Macadamia nuts Pine nuts Almonds
Meat	Beef
Sweeteners	Cane sugar, sorghum, corn syrup, glucose, dextrose
Beverages	Tea: Sassafras tea or papaya leaf tea, mate tea, lemon verbena tea Milk Juices may be made and used without added sweeteners from the fruits and vegetables listed above in any combination desired
Soup	May be made from any of the above ingredients—meat, vegetables, and spices
Miscellaneous	Milk products: Butter, cheese, oleomargarine (without coloring), yogurt

Miscellaneous (cont)	Corn oil
	Mushrooms and yeast (brewer's yeast, etc.)
	Vanilla

Tips related to the rotary diet

· It may take three weeks for benefit to be noted on a rotary diet. Don't get discouraged. After the first few days, it becomes much easier to plan and adjust to this new way of eating.

· Don't eat any food, even if it is listed, if you know it causes you to become ill. Even though it says, for example, that eggs are an allowed food on day one, you can't eat them if they make you sick.

· If you are, for example, wheat sensitive, you may be able to tolerate wheat once a day, every four days. If you eat too much, too often, you may not improve on the diet. In time, if you adhere to the diet, you may be able to eat your problem foods more than once a day, and more often than every four days.

· Start with a few foods allowed on each specific day. Later on, if you seem fine on that day, gradually expand the number of foods you are eating.

· Start with only one food in a family list. Expand within each family, only if the first food is all right. Example: start with orange and if that causes no symptoms, you may try grapefruit, etc.

· If a reaction occurs to some food, try bicarbonate. Use your physician's medication or those listed in the "Special Tips" section above.

· Use fruit with water or fruit juice on cereal, if no milk is allowed on a certain day. For soda pop, use fruit juice and carbonated water.

· The rotary diet can be adapted for any age group. A young infant may eat only one or two foods from each of the four-day lists. Gradually, new foods can be added one at a time.

· A nursing mother with an ill infant may have to place herself and the infant on the rotary diet to find out what is bothering the baby. The foods a mother eats may be found in her milk.

· If you don't want to eat a food on a list, don't eat it.

· If you want to change something from one day to another, it is all right, but you must not eat any food more often than every four days. You also must keep beef and milk, and egg and chicken on the same days.

· If you substitute honey in a recipe, use the same amount of honey as sugar. For example, 1 cup honey = 1 cup sugar or 1 cup of maple sugar or ¾ cup molasses plus ¼ tsp. soda. If you want items less sweet, use ½ cup honey for 1 cup sugar. Honey is a liquid, so you must decrease the liquid in the recipe by ¼ cup. For example, change 1 cup milk to ¾ cup milk, so the batter consistency is correct (Dworkin and Dworkin 1974).

· Cellu Cereal-Free Baking Powder is available at health food stores.

· One cup butter = ⅞ cup oil (not recommended for cookies).

· If your child cannot drink milk or soymilk, be certain to check about the need for calcium with your physician (see appendix B5).

· No prepackaged foods with additives and preservatives are allowed on this diet. Visit a health food store for cereal or flour.

· All grains are purposely placed on day four of the diet rotation. If you try each one separately at four-day intervals on several occasions and notice no adverse effect, you may then try to use rice on day one, oats or barley on day two, and wheat on day three, leaving corn and rye for day four. Some patients, however, are so grain sensitive that they cannot tolerate any grain more often than every four days.

· If you can't find some of the items listed, try a health food store.

If a food always causes a digestive problem, is it allergy?

Of course not. Common examples are the following:

· Prunes and baked beans often cause loose bowel movements or belly gas.

· Corn often passes undigested through the intestines.

· Some families seem to lack enzymes so they cannot eat greasy foods.

· Some families lack enzymes to dissolve milk sugars, so milk causes diarrhea.

· Improperly canned foods may contain bacteria which cause illness.

· Greasy, foamy, frothy bowel movements may indicate fibrocystic disease.

· Infant feeding problems are sometimes due to a food allergy, but often they are due to an improper formula temperature, nipple holes which are too small or large, or improper positioning of the infant during feeding.

Your physician can help you decide if your child's digestive problems are or are not allergy.

You've tried diets before and they didn't help?

There are ways and ways to diet. If a physician tells you milk may be a problem and you stop drinking milk and don't get better, it does not mean milk is all right. You can't assume milk is not at fault unless you remained ill after not eating or drinking a speck of anything which contained milk for about two weeks. Check diet lists in Appendix B for uncommon locations for foods. Few people would know milk is in luncheon meat, some baby fruit desserts such as banana, in most soups and some bread. You must read labels, not make mistakes and follow the diet for an adequate period of time or you can't conclude a food is not a problem.

Some people appear to have some basic overwhelming problem which appears to make them react to many foods. If you are sensitive to milk, wheat, and eggs, even though you stop all milk, your health may not improve because you are still eating wheat and egg. For complicated food problems seek an allergist or physician who is knowledgeable and successful in the detection and treatment of food problems (see appendix C3).

Are there any special cautions about food allergy which need repeating?

Yes, two main ones.

· Never give anyone in your family a food which you know causes a severe allergic reaction. It might be very harmful.

· Although parents' or patients' observations are often correct, valid interpretation may be obscure or require specialized training or knowledge. A simple example is the effect noted after someone drinks an excess of Scotch and water, bourbon and water, or vodka and water. We all know water is not causing the symptoms. Less obvious examples, however, are symptoms caused by dye or flavor in toothpaste, wheat in soup, or egg white in mayonnaise or some types of root beer.

Are all food problems or sensitivities a food allergy?

Of course not. Food problems can be due to multiple body malfunctions which are entirely unrelated to allergy. The big question and controversy revolves around the scope and extent of food allergy as a cause of disease in our society. Von Pirquet, in 1906, coined the term allergy to denote an altered reactivity resulting from repeated exposure to antigenic or infective substances. Unfortunately, the present-day definition has changed and is not employed consistently (Dohan and Grasberger 1973). Some allergists recognize only a restricted immunologic definition of food allergy. They believe only a small percentage, maybe 5 to 10 percent of the population, are so affected. To these allergists, a food allergy reaction must occur after ingestion of a minute amount of food and symptoms must occur within a few minutes after ingestion. The patient must also have a special type of antibody called immunoglobulin E (IgE) directed against that specific food. In addition, the reaction must cause symptoms only in specified parts of the body. For example, an immediate reaction to a nut, fish, or egg is accepted by all allergists as a possible cause of hives, body swelling, hay fever-like symptoms, asthma, or intestinal complaints.

Physicians, however, who use a less restricted definition of food allergy, believe that as many as 70 percent of the population may have this problem. They have observed foods to cause the identical reactions, in identical body parts as mentioned previously, but the symptoms may not occur until several hours after ingestion. They believe that virtually any area of the body may be affected by altered reactivity. For example, if a child develops asthma and hyperactivity after drinking milk, is the asthma an allergy, while hyperactivity is not?

They believe there may be immunological or other mechanisms, which are not presently understood, to explain not only adverse reactions to a food, but also, the associated favorable response noted after oral or injection food treatment (see chapter 4). All the mechanisms related to food problems are not known and simply cannot be explained by our present storehouse of immunologic and other medical data. While such knowledge is desirable and necessary for proper understanding, it is not essential for practical application. The important fact is: If someone stops eating a food, does he feel well? If he eats a certain food, will he become ill? If food avoidance solves the problem and does not harm the patient, this is the essence of the practice of medicine. Time alone will tell if the current (limited) or the original (less restricted) definition of food allergy will prove to be correct. In the meantime, we can surely wait a while to understand the hows and whys, whether we call it a food problem, idiosyncrasy, sensitivity, intolerance, or allergy.

4 · Will a One-Week Diet Help?

This chapter tells you in detail exactly how to do a one-week diet which omits major foods or dyes commonly thought to affect activity and behavior in children. Tips to prevent diet errors are given. It explains some diet shortcuts which may give answers more quickly. It tells how to detect additional unsuspected food offenders. It candidly discusses possible avenues for treating single or multiple food problems. It details what you can do if the diet fails. Some illustrative case histories are given.

A one-week diet to help patients who have hyperactivity, fatigue, or behavior or learning problems is detailed in appendix B3. In addition, any patient who has some of the many common or atypical possible symptoms of allergy listed in the chapter 3 checklists might also be helped.

Before you do the diet, fill in the "Hyperkinesis Parent's Questionnaire" in chapter 2. By comparing the medical problems and activity scores before the diet with those after the diet, you may be able to evaluate more accurately how much your child (or family) has been helped.

Considerations to be made before you start the diet

Discuss the diet with your child before you begin, if your child is old enough to understand what is being done. Don't just tell your child he must go on the diet because you want to see if it will help him. Instead, ask him if he would like to try a one-week diet. Explain, in terms he will understand, why he would want to try it. What is it that he misses most or can't do or have because he is too active or has learning or behavior problems? Discuss the diet in terms of what he has to gain if he is fully cooperative. Most children desperately want to be helped and, with the proper approach, they will enthusiastically begin the diet. Stress that the diet usually takes only a week, and then favorite foods can be eaten again. Explain that the second week of the diet will be the fun part. There will be a chocolate day, a sugar day, a milk day, and so on. Mark these days on the calendar so he can follow the countdown until he can eat what he likes again. Offer a reward if he follows the diet to the letter. Stress, however, that accidents can occur and if he makes a mistake, he must be sure to tell you so you can properly evaluate the value of the diet. Let your child help with as much of the diet planning as possible. Be positive, but honest and realistic. Do not guarantee success, but explain that children who have problems similar to his have sometimes been helped.

The diet can be tried while your child is taking medicine

Ritalin or similar drugs can be continued during the diet if desired. If, however, you don't see much difference whether the drugs are taken or not, talk to your physician about stopping the drugs temporarily, or using them only if they are needed. Most children forget to take their drugs occasionally, even if they know medicine is necessary. Parents easily recognize missed doses. If you find, however, after your child has dieted for several days, a missed dose of medicine is no longer noticeable, you may have found the answer to your child's problem.

While some children appear to be able to discontinue their activity-modifying drugs during the diet, others continue to need the same or a lower dose of medication. All children, however, who continue to require medication are not diet failures. Some parents find that either the diet or the drugs help a little, but by using both at the same time, their child improves to a greater degree than ever before.

Other medicines, such as those for asthma or hay fever, should not be continued during the diet unless definitely needed. Check with your physician. These medicines may contain food coloring, sugar, and corn. Some children are so sensitive that the small amount of these items in medicine can cause symptoms. Don't start the diet if your child is on an antibiotic. Wait until the infection is gone.

Dangers of the diet

There are a few. If your child has a known allergy to some food in the diet, don't feed it to your child. If your child has asthma, be careful when you re-add foods to your child's diet. If someone doesn't eat a food for several days, when it is eaten again, it can sometimes cause a dramatic, exaggerated reaction. This could cause an alarming problem for some asthmatics. Be sure you have medicine to treat asthma and check with your physician before you begin the diet (see chapter 3). If you find that your child is sensitive to several frequently eaten foods, you must not continue the diet for over two weeks without supervision. You must check with your physician if you want to avoid any of the food items tested for a prolonged period of time. Avoidance of some foods in children or adults can lead to nutritional problems. For example, if your child drinks no milk or only soybean milk, a deficiency of calcium might lead to improper bone growth. Your physician can advise which of several preparations to use. Neo-Calglucon Syrup or chewable Di-Cal-D wafers or tablets are only two of many types available (see appendix B5).

HOW TO DO THE DIET

First, read this chapter completely a couple of times so you can understand as much as possible before you begin. In this way, common errors might be avoided. The diet is in four major parts.

· *The Diet Part.* A number of common suspect foods are not eaten.

· *The Answer Part.* Each suspect food is eaten, one at a time, to see if any cause symptoms.

· *The Confirmation Part.* Each suspect food is tested again to confirm if it really causes symptoms.

· *The Decision Part.* How is the food problem to be treated: Avoidance, drugs, or food therapy?

The diet part

Your child will be allowed to eat only specified meats, fruit, and vegetables for one full week. No milk, wheat, egg, cocoa, sugar,

corn, or food coloring is allowed. During this period, it is absolutely essential that you keep exact records of everything your
child eats during the entire week (see appendix B2). It is possible
that you might need this information later on, so take the time to
record everything.

Select a time when your home life looks rather calm and
organized for about two weeks. Place your child or affected family
members on the diet in appendix B3. Recipes to make it easier and
more pleasant are in appendix B4. Some children may seem better
in a couple of days or within a week. A few children might not
improve for two weeks. Sometimes there is no improvement.

Do the diet once and try very hard to do it correctly. Of course
you will make mistakes, but if you or your child make too many
errors, the diet may not help, even if one of the foods being investigated is the cause of the problem.

If your child is the same or worse after the one-week diet, skip
ahead to "The Diet Helped a Little, or Not at All." If your child
improved on the diet—read on.

The answer part

If your child is a little or much better on the diet, we must figure
out which food items might be at fault. During the second week,
therefore, each of the possible offending foods—milk, wheat, egg,
cocoa, sugar, corn, and food coloring—are added back into the
diet. One food item is reintroduced each day. When a suspect food
is eaten again, your child should be encouraged to eat as much of it
as possible. We want to see what happens.

For example, suppose your child was on the one-week diet from
Sunday through Saturday. The next day, Sunday, give your child
tremendous quantities of milk and dairy products; on Monday, add
wheat or flour; on Tuesday, add sugar; on Wednesday, eggs; on
Thursday, chocolate; on Friday, dyed foods; and on Saturday, corn
products. The record sheet in appendix B2 will help with this portion of the diet study. It is easier if the foods are added back in the
order just outlined. You may find that one food causes your child to
become hyperactive, another may cause a bellyache, and a third, a
stuffy nose and a behavior problem. Don't guess. Wait and see
what happens.

There are a number of tips which will make the addition of foods
back into your child's diet easier. The following suggestions will
help with each food. If you already know that one of the foods in

the diet study causes an alarming or severe reaction, don't check that food. If you are in doubt, check with your physician.

Sunday—Milk Day

Give your child a large quantity of milk, whipped cream sweetened with saccharin, sucaryl, or pure honey, and cottage cheese. Butter, margarine, and yellow cheese are not allowed unless you are absolutely certain they don't contain yellow dye. Do not allow ice cream, because it contains many items that might cause symptoms. If your child has symptoms within an hour or anytime on Sunday or early Monday morning before eating, milk may be a problem and should be avoided in all forms. Appendix B5 tells exactly which foods do and do not contain milk or dairy products.

Monday—Wheat Day

Give your child plain soda crackers or pure wheat cereal (health food store) or Wheatena. If milk was no problem on Sunday, milk on cereal and cottage cheese and noncolored dairy products are allowed. If milk caused symptoms, however, continue to avoid all products that contain milk in any form (see appendix B5). A natural, unsweetened fruit juice which contains no artificial coloring, such as Welch's bottled grape juice, Dole unsweetened pineapple juice, or Minute Maid orange juice can replace milk on cereal, if necessary. See appendix B6 for foods which do and do not contain wheat.

Tuesday—Sugar Day

Give your child sugar cubes and add granulated sugar to all allowed foods. Be sure the sugar given is the usual sugar you use. It is possible to be sensitive to only certain types—that is, beet, corn, cane, etc. If milk and wheat caused no symptoms on Sunday or Monday, these foods may continue to be eaten.

If, however, milk or wheat caused difficulty, continue to avoid the offending food item in all forms. If your child ingests milk and wheat when one or both causes symptoms, you won't be able to tell what effect sugar has on your child when this is also eaten. See appendix B7 for foods which do and do not contain sugar.

Wednesday—Egg Day

Add eggs in their usual form, cooked or as an egg nog. Give custard. Remember, if sugar was a problem no egg item which contains sugar can be given. If wheat caused symptoms, no toast. If milk was a problem, no butter or milk can be used in eggs which are eaten. See appendix B8 for foods which do and do not contain eggs.

Thursday—Chocolate Day

On this day, eat dark chocolate and cocoa. Milk chocolate can't be eaten unless there was no trouble with sugar or milk. Hot chocolate can be made with hot water, Hershey's cocoa powder, pure honey, or an artificial sweetener. Don't eat candy bars because most contain corn. Don't eat foods that contain eggs if eggs caused symptoms.

If milk, wheat, and eggs did not cause symptoms, you can bake a chocolate cake or cookies. Use Crisco, lard, or oil for baking if dyes in butter or margarine are a problem. See appendix B9 for foods which do and do not contain chocolate.

Friday—Food Coloring Day

If sugar caused no difficulty, give your child Jell-O, jelly, and artificially-colored fruit beverages, such as soda pop and Kool-Aid or popsicles. If wheat was all right, your child also may have artificially colored wheat cereal. Try to give as many yellow, orange, green, purple, and red food items as possible, because only one color might cause symptoms.

If sugar caused symptoms on Tuesday, your child can only eat items which contain no sugar. The dyed foods must be sweetened with pure honey, saccharin or Sucaryl. You can buy dietetic pop or gelatin (D'Zerta). If milk or wheat caused symptoms, continue to avoid them. See appendix B10 for foods which do and do not contain food coloring.

Saturday—Corn Day

Feed your child whole kernel corn, corn meal, corn flakes, and popcorn. You cannot use milk on cereal or butter on popcorn if milk caused symptoms. If sugar was a problem, use pure honey or saccharin. If food coloring was a problem, don't use butter or margarine. Natural fruit juice, which is not colored (Dole's pineapple, Minute Maid orange, or bottled Welch's grape), can be used on cereal. Popcorn can be made with sea salt and liquified Crisco or safflower oil if necessary. See appendix B11 for foods which do and do not contain corn.

One or More Foods Caused a Reaction. If a food causes a reaction, it often happens within an hour if the food has not been eaten for five to ten days. Sometimes, however, the reaction may not occur until late in the evening, during the night or the next morning. If a reaction definitely occurs, give your child a bicarbonate preparation, such as Alka-Seltzer Antacid Formula without Aspirin.

Possible Problems. There are relatively few problems when children are placed on the one-week diet. If the child eats only what is allowed, parents readily can see if the diet helps or not. A few will be better in two or three days, but most will not be helped for about a week.

Problems sometimes arise during the second part of the diet-study period when foods are re-added. These tips may help.

· Your child has finished the first part of the one-week diet and seems better. The very morning you are to add the first food (milk), your child has a bellyache, is extremely hyperactive, or seems unwell because of a cold or an infection. Don't add the food! You must wait until he is his "usual" self again. Add milk on Monday or Tuesday, not Sunday, and add each of the remaining foods a day or two later than planned. Stay on the original diet a few extra days.

· Your child eats one of the test foods in large amounts. Within an hour he is obviously hyperactive, a behavior problem, has a bellyache, or other problems. Give Alka-Seltzer Antacid Formula without Aspirin. It might help. Don't give any more of the food that appeared to cause the symptoms. See appendix B for unsuspected hidden forms of the food which must be avoided. From this occurrence, you can be suspicious about this food, but it is only a suspicion.

· You feed your child milk (or any of the other test foods) and he has a definite reaction which begins within an hour or later in the day. The reaction, however, doesn't stop in a little while, but lasts through that day, and the next morning he is still having difficulty. Do you add the next food? No. If you add wheat while your child is still reacting to milk, you can't tell what is going on. Wait until the milk reaction is gone and he is normal (for him). Then add wheat and the remaining foods a day or so later than expected. It is possible for a reaction to one food to last for two to four days, but most reactions start and stop within a few hours.

· Your child won't take Alka-Seltzer Antacid Formula without Aspirin or any bicarbonate preparation. What should you do? If he won't take it, try to put it secretly into some liquid other than water. De-fizz it completely before your child drinks it. Sometimes a child will take it if it is hidden in Welch's bottled grape juice or Minute Maid orange juice. If Alka-Seltzer Antacid Formula without Aspirin causes a bellyache, be sure your child drinks at least one large glass of liquid after it is taken.

· Your child may take Alka-Seltzer Antacid Formula without Aspirin and not be helped. This can happen; it doesn't help everyone.

· If something special (a picnic, party, etc.) occurs during the period when you are re-adding foods, don't re-add any food on that day. Merely keep the child on the original one-week diet plus any foods that you already checked and found to be all right. If, for example, you add sugar on the day your child is going to a school party, if he becomes hyperactive, how can you tell if it was the sugar or something else that he ate on that day?

· Check the record lists you've kept of the exact foods your child ate when he was on the one-week diet and also when you re-added the suspicious foods back into the diet. If your child reacted on a certain day, it might not be the food you added back into the diet, but some other food which caused trouble. With these lists, your doctor can help you figure out which other food might be causing the trouble. For example, suppose your child eats peanut butter on the day you checked to see if sugar is a problem. He has symptoms. In five to ten days when you recheck sugar he is all right. If you have a record that he ate peanut butter the first time sugar was tested, but not the second time, it may help you realize that you now have to check peanut butter. You can check any food to see if it causes symptoms by giving a lot of it on the fifth day. If your child repeatedly has symptoms on the fifth day, you have one answer.

· Don't try to add foods back into the diet if your child will not be home. Add a food, for example, when your child comes home from school or on a weekend, but not ten minutes before he catches the school bus. If he is staying with a friend or relative at night, or is out every evening, you can't tell what effect the food had. The teacher can help tell you how he is when he is at school, but you may have to call her each day. Don't influence her. Merely say you are trying different things to see how they affect your child's activity and did your child seem the same, better, or worse today? If he really gets bad, she will know it.

· Your child develops a fever or serious infection when you are trying to do the diet. What can you do? Wait until the infection is over and start all over again. Most liquid medicines and colored tablets are dyed and sweetened, and most tablets contain corn. Some people are so sensitive that the little bit of dye, corn, and sugar in the medicine can cause symptoms.

· Everybody makes mistakes and with diet studies it is sure to happen. If something is eaten by mistake, do not be concerned if nothing happens. If a reaction occurs, however, when you've added one food on purpose and one by mistake, stop everything until the reaction is over and then recheck these two items, one at a time, at five-day intervals.

To Determine Which Specific Food Coloring Is Causing Trouble. The following method can be used to detect which food coloring causes your child to have a reaction. Remember, however, that bottles of food coloring in grocery stores or artificially colored foods or beverages often contain a mixture of a number of dyes to make each color. For example, one gelatin dessert might be one shade of red because of two red dyes, while another is a different shade because of two other red dyes. It is therefore possible for your child to react to some red items but not to others. The same is also true for other colors.

Do *not* do the following test unless your child appears to be able to eat foods that are artificially colored without any difficulty. The easiest way to check for grocery-store food coloring is to place one or two drops of red under your child's tongue and have him silently count slowly to sixty before swallowing. Casually observe your child for about twenty minutes. Don't let him eat during this period of time. Does he change? If he does, see if Alka-Seltzer Antacid Formula without Aspirin helps. If the latter does not help, you will have to wait until the reaction stops, but at least you know a red food dye is suspect (see appendix B10). If there is no change, red may not be the problem, but you will have to repeat the test using yellow and then blue coloring.

If you find red is a problem, any item that is red, purple, or orange may cause symptoms. If you find yellow causes symptoms, any green, yellow, or orange item could cause trouble. If you find blue a problem, watch blue, green, and purple foods, beverages, medicines, and pills.

Remember, if food coloring is your child's problem, it may be almost impossible to avoid dyes, because many foods are not adequately labeled. Fresh frozen or canned items may contain dyes and this may not be indicated on the label. To further complicate the problem, some items like Coffee Rich, which appear white may contain yellow dye (see "Food Coloring" in appendix E4).

The Confirmation Part

You finally have the answer. By using the one-week diet, you found which symptoms were eliminated in part or completely. By re-adding foods, one at a time, you suspect which foods appear to cause specific undesirable symptoms. Now what do you do?

Recheck the foods in question first. It may be a coincidence that your child got worse the day you added a food back into the diet. First, give your child the food in question again for one day, then stop that food in all forms (see individual food diet lists) for five days to ten days. Then feed your child a large amount of the food being tested for at least one or two days. If a similar reaction does not occur when the food is eaten the second time, be skeptical. That food may not be a problem. If there is still some doubt, recheck a third time.

You can come to the wrong conclusion if your child ate lots of the food the first time and very little the next two times. You also can be fooled if the first time, the food was eaten only on the specified first and fifth day, but, the second and third times, a little of the food was eaten almost every day for five days. Try to repeat the tests as carefully as possible. For a number of reasons, if you eat a food every day, you may not realize it is causing symptoms. If you totally avoid a food for several weeks, when you add it back, you may not realize it is a problem because the symptoms return so gradually you don't recognize the relation between the food and symptoms. The key is to eat a suspect food only at a five- to ten-day interval.

One reason food sensitivities are so seldom diagnosed is that they are not easy to figure out. It takes time and thought. Even if you do everything correctly, you can be fooled. For example, suppose you eat bread in excess and then avoid it for four full days. When you eat it again, you may have definite symptoms within an hour, so you assume wheat is your problem. However, it may be yeast or preservatives in the flour. It might be insecticides which happen to be left in the grain after storage. The egg white that is put on the crust of a loaf of bread to make it shiny might be the problem. You should merely try to figure out which food items appear to cause symptoms. Your physician can be the super sleuth to help you determine which component or unsuspected food contaminant might be causing symptoms.

The Decision Part

You know which foods are problems. Decision time has come. You must decide which alternative course you choose to follow. Your choices include diet, drugs, or food treatment. Each has certain advantages and disadvantages. You have to decide which is best for your child and for your family.

Diet. The advantages of total elimination of offending foods from your child's diet is that it quickly and inexpensively eliminates the problem. You have taken the nails from the shoe and by eliminating the cause, symptoms should no longer be evident. After three to six months, some of the foods which initially had to be eliminated totally from the diet often can be eaten every five days without difficulty. Special cookbooks related to allergy make dieting easier and more pleasant (see appendix C4).

The disadvantages of a diet, to a degree, depend upon which foods have to be avoided. Egg, chocolate, and dyed foods are difficult, but possible to avoid. Milk, wheat, sugar, and corn are major challenges. Sometimes a food sensitivity is so strong, it persists no matter how long the food is avoided. This is called a fixed food allergy. It will not be outgrown. Sometimes parents find they can compromise by limiting certain foods as much as possible when their child is home. A little of the problem-food items eaten in school or for special occasions may be tolerated. If offending foods, however, are eaten too often or in large amounts, the sensitivity may increase, necessitating total abstinence. Trial and error will quickly show parents and children how often and how much of which food items can be tolerated.

If a stringent diet must be followed for a prolonged time, a physician must monitor the patient's nutrition. This is true for adults, as well as growing children.

Drugs. Some parents decide they want no part of any diet. Both parents work and the child may have a busy social or sports schedule. For innumerable reasons, it is impossible to adhere sufficiently to a diet to make it helpful. If a drug such as Ritalin helps your child, this indeed may be the best way to treat your particular child's hyperactivity.

Problems arise, however, if none of the usual drugs relieve your child's symptoms sufficiently or if side effects from an effective drug cause intolerable symptoms (see chapter 2).

A new drug called cromolyn, sold by prescription under the names of Aarane or Intal, is effective in preventing and treating asthma. Approximately 85 percent of this drug enters the intestinal tract when the white powder is inhaled through the mouth into the lungs. Preliminary research studies in 1977 suggest that diverse food-allergy symptoms also may be relieved by this drug, if the cromolyn powder is dissolved in water and swallowed twenty minutes before eating foods which cause known allergy (Nizami et al. 1977). This drug seems, in some instances, to effectively reduce or eliminate the adverse symptoms caused by offending foods. At present studies are still being conducted in relation to the effect of cromolyn on hyperactivity (Simeon et al. 1978). During the next year or so these may determine if cromolyn is an alternate form of drug therapy which may allow a patient to eat offending foods without the latter causing symptoms.

Food Treatment. The advantage of this method is that it, literally, allows you to have your cake and eat it too. With food therapy, most offending foods can be ingested in moderation without causing symptoms. In addition, methods used to treat food allergy also can be used diagnostically to determine which foods cause symptoms, so diets may be unnecessary.

The major disadvantage of food therapy is that the effectiveness of this method of treatment has not been confirmed scientifically to the satisfaction of many allergists (Breneman 1973, Crawford 1976). Only ecologists and a minority of allergists, otolaryngologists, pediatricians, and general practitioners know how to test and treat food problems effectively (see appendix C3). As with many techniques used in medicine, success is determined not by *what* is done, but by how it is done. Improper application and evaluation of the nuances of this new method for diagnosis and treatment can lead to spurious impressions and conclusions. Fortunately, the safety of food therapy is not in question because extracts or solutions used for food treatment are essentially the same as have been used for years to test and treat pollen or other types of common allergy.

FOOD TESTING AND TREATMENT

Standard food-allergy extract solutions are used for testing after a series of 1:5 dilutions are prepared. The doctor may test the patient by placing certain dilutions of foods under the tongue (sublingual testing) or by injecting tiny amounts of extract into the skin (intradermal testing). Some dilutions of foods appear to cause symptoms, for example, hyperactivity, bellyaches, or a stuffy nose, while other dilutions appear to relieve these same symptoms. Patients are then treated either sublingually (Morris 1969, Green 1974, Hawley and Buckley 1974a, b, Dickey 1971b, 1976a, b, Rapp 1978a, b, c, d), or by subcutaneous injections (Black 1942, Willoughby 1974, Miller 1977) with the exact dilution of a food which appears to relieve or stop their symptoms during diagnostic testing sessions. If a patient has numerous food sensitivities, correct treatment dilutions of several foods can be combined.

In general, sublingual food therapy is needed three times a day at first, but in time the need slowly decreases to twice a week. Subcutaneous food therapy is initially needed on a daily basis, but in a very few weeks, treatments may be needed only once or twice a week.

Although sublingual therapy is obviously preferred, it is not as helpful as subcutaneous therapy for some patients. Many who have food problems appear to be helped by either form of therapy. A favorable response is often noted after once major offending foods are treated. Some hyperactive children also require a treatment with dust, molds, or other items that commonly cause allergy.

How parents can evaluate the effectiveness of food therapy

If you know that each time your child eats a food he becomes hyperactive or has other symptoms, it is easy to determine if food treatment helps. Purposely feed your child the offending food, wait for symptoms to develop. Does sublingual or subcutaneous food therapy relieve the problem? Another method is to give the food treatment before the food is eaten and notice if symptoms repeatedly can be prevented.

Once a patient is well treated, it is not unusual for a parent to forget to give food therapy. When symptoms arise, does reinstitution of therapy help? If an excessive amount of an offending food is ingested, symptoms often recur. These should readily subside after additional food therapy. At any point, a parent can discontinue therapy and notice if food symptoms recur. If they do, food therapy should give relief.

Some parents want their child to be helped so much that they see improvement when it isn't there. Similarly, a child may want to eat a food so badly that he says food treatment helps, when it does not. If food treatment is truly effective, your child's activity score will decrease, his symptoms will obviously lessen and friends, relatives, neighbors, and teachers will notice improvement. The improvement won't last for a week or two, but for a prolonged period of time.

Parents sometimes may be fooled if a child develops a new food problem. For example, suppose a child is not treated for peanut butter, but develops a craving for it and then becomes sensitive to it. If his food therapy does not contain peanut, it obviously won't relieve symptoms due to peanut. If a bicarbonate preparation relieves the symptoms when food therapy fails this may indicate a missed food problem. Give your physician a detailed list of foods your child ate for the twelve-hour period prior to the onset of symptoms, and he will help you determine if peanut or some other food is at fault.

Another source of confusion is a changed food-treatment dose. Suppose milk causes no difficulty for several months providing sublingual milk drops are taken regularly. Then you notice milk causes symptoms in spite of milk treatment. It may indicate the physician needs to determine a new treatment dosage for milk. A few patients seem particularly prone to this type of problem. Fortunately, most patients only infrequently need changes in their food treatment.

One last source of difficulty is noted when a patient tries to use food therapy less often. If sublingual drops are used three times a day for several weeks, it is often possible to lower the dose to twice a day. Some patients are in a rush, however, and suddenly switch from three times a day to once every other day, so symptoms recur. If food treatment is taken more often, this readily solves this problem.

Scientific study of food therapy

For many years, the only way to treat food allergy was to stop eating the problem food. In search of a better way, however, at the turn of this century, pioneer physicians began to feed patients weak solutions of foods (Schofield 1908, Schloss 1912, Cooke 1922). As the solutions were gradually made stronger, it was noted that some patients could eat some of the foods which had previously caused illness. In 1935, Drs. Keston, Waters, and Hopkins reported successful food treatment in fifty patients with eczema. In 1942, Dr. Harvey Black, co-author of the major allergy text used by physicians until the middle of this century, published an article validating the effectiveness of food therapy. He first confirmed the patients' history by purposely feeding them foods known to cause asthma. As a control, patients also were fed other foods to show these did not cause wheezing. He treated one hundred of his patients with gradually stronger solutions of specific foods to which they were sensitive until the wheezing subsided. Another fifty patients merely avoided their problem foods. After five months, all patients were again fed their offending foods. No asthma was noted in 73 percent of treated patients, while 12 percent of untreated patients improved. This indicates that about 12 percent of patients appear to "outgrow" their food allergy, but with food treatment, an additional 60 percent appear to improve.

In 1961, Dr. Carlton Lee attempted to find a better means to treat food problems because both he and his wife had severe food allergies. His studies, as well as those of Dr. H. Rinkel, revealed that solutions of offending foods caused symptoms if they were either too strong or too weak. When the correct strength solution, however, was used for therapy, it was possible to eat many offending foods. Over the years, a number of variations of his original methods have been suggested (Rinkel et al. 1964, Lee et al. 1969, Morris 1969, Willoughby 1974, Miller 1977). It appears that some patients can obtain relief if the correct dosage and dilution of food is administered under the tongue or subcutaneously. A possible reason why some earlier investigations concerning food treatment were unsuccessful could be related to a lack of training or skill in the determination of the correct strength of food solution to use for therapy. This may also help explain why two collaborative studies have indicated food therapy is ineffective (Breneman et al. 1973, Crawford 1976).

Recent well-documented studies by experienced clinical ecologists, many of which have been double blind, confirm the efficacy of new methods for the detection and/or treatment of food sensitivities (Green 1974, Rea 1976, 1977, Morris 1969, Miller 1977, Sandberg et al. 1977, Rapp 1978a, b, c, d). Ecologists have adopted many suggestions by earlier investigators, especially those of Dr. T. Randolph, to combat food problems. Individualized patient care often includes a combination of food restriction, a rotary diet, food therapy, and stringent avoidance of known chemical offenders. These physicians are seriously concerned about health problems related to the ever-increasing pollution and contamination of our food, water, air, and homes. They stress relief of chronic symptoms by elimination of causative factors, rather than drug therapy.

Why food therapy helps

We do not know. Our present state of knowledge cannot explain why one dilution of a food appears to cause symptoms while another dilution, often weaker, relieves symptoms. The observation is easily confirmed, but not easily explained. It is not unusual, however, to know how to relieve a patient's symptoms long before medical-research scientists can explain why such therapy is effective.

THE DIET HELPED A LITTLE, OR NOT AT ALL

The following tips may aid parents who found only partial improvement in their child's activity during the diet. Some children's hyperactivity will not be relieved in any way by the one-week diet. Sometimes, although bellyaches, nose symptoms, or behavior problems improve, activity is not helped. Here are a few reasons why the one-week diet might fail.

· Your child might need a two-week diet. Some children do not improve until the tenth to fourteenth day. Check with your physician if you want to try a longer diet (see "Stephen" in chapter 1).

· You tried the one-week diet, but it was not done correctly. Most mistakes are misunderstandings. Common errors include: (1) Failure to adhere to the diet. Check your diet records. Were *only* the allowed foods eaten? Did you read *all* food labels? (2) Failure to appreciate that some children can be so sensitive to some foods that the odor of a food can cause symptoms. Eggs, fish, nuts, peanut butter, potatoes, corn, and buckwheat odors are known to cause symptoms in some patients. If you allowed your child to eat a little of the forbidden foods, that little bit might have been too much.

· Prepackaged foods are not only sometimes deceptively labeled, but in many instances, the exact ingredients are entirely omitted from the label. For example, milk may be called sodium caseinate or whey on a label, or, if the amount of milk in a food is tiny, the container may not state that it contains milk.

· Your child may be sensitive to some foods excluded in the one-week diet, as well as a few other foods. This could account for a total lack of improvement or partial help from the one-week diet. Other common foods which may alter a child's activity include any form of oranges, grapes, apples, peanuts, beef, or tomatoes. Try omitting each additional suspect food as suggested above. Children with multiple sensitivities may require the aid of a physician who is knowledgeable and successful in treating food problems (see appendix C3).

· Your child may need a different diet. See Dr. Crook's food diet (appendix B18) or Dr. Feingold's diet, which excludes artificial food coloring, artificial flavoring, and natural salicylates (appendix B16). If your child improves on either of these diets, re-add one food at a time. Try single foods, such as peaches, beef, and so on, but not mixtures, such as spaghetti or vegetable soup, so you can readily detect offending items.

· More and more evidence points to preservatives and food additives as possible causes of increased activity and other symptoms in children (see appendix B17). Common ones are the antioxidants, BHT (butylated hydroxytoluene) and BHA (butylated hydroxyanisole); others include buffers, emulsifiers, flavorings, sequestrants, minerals, neutralizing substances, preservatives, pesticides, stabilizers or thickeners, sweetening agents, bleaching agents, or vitamins. Try strict avoidance of all these items for two full weeks.

· Some children become hyperactive after exposure to odors or contacts of the types listed by Kailin and Brooks (1963) and appendixes E 2, 3, and 4.

· Common items within a home which can cause difficulty are listed throughout Appendix E, which also provides details on exactly how to make your home more allergy and/or chemical free.

· Some children are definitely more active or develop behavior problems during pollen or mold-spore seasons. See Appendix D for pollen seasons in your area of the United States. Appropriate injection treatment may relieve this type of hyperactivity.

· Some hyperactivity appears to be related to contact with molds in a home, or on or in foods. See appendix D2 for discussion of how to recognize and cope with this problem. Treatment for mold sensitivity appears to relieve symptoms of hyperactivity in some children.

· Hyperactivity can be related to many medical problems entirely unrelated to the inside or outside of your home or to foods. These problems are discussed in chapter 2. Some children have more than one reason for their increased activity.

· Years of hyperactivity with associated behavior and learning problems can cause chronic, detrimental patterns of reaction within a family or in social settings which require modification through family counseling. Once the child is more quiet, he and his family are more responsive and able to take positive strides to resolve major residual, interpersonal problems.

Here are a few examples of why the one-week diet did not help.

J. G., a seven-year-old white male, was placed on the diet. Although his activity became normal within one week, his behavior did not improve. He finally had to be placed on Ritalin, solely to help his behavior. His mother found if he did not eat any sugar, his activity was normal but his behavior remained a problem. There are several possible answers. The behavior problem may be entirely unrelated to the foods excluded in the diet. Foods which were not tested or some other home or family factors, odors, contacts, molds or pollens might be at fault. The behavior problem may be related to other medical problems (see chapter 2). His mother must record contacts and foods eaten on days when he is fine and compare these with similar bad-day records (see chapter 3).

Another seven-year-old boy, P. L., had been hyperactive since birth. He had year-round nose allergies, headaches once a week, frequent bellyaches, crying spells, depression, excessive talking, irritability, and constant wiggling. In less than a week, while on the diet, he no longer had abdominal complaints or headaches; his nose and disposition were better, but his activity was entirely unchanged. He was placed on a strict Feingold diet and within a week, he was moderately better. His mother allowed him to eat individual foods which were omitted from the Feingold diet, one at a time, and found that twenty minutes after he drank tea he was markedly active. After avoiding tea, for the first time, he could sit still and not wiggle his hands and feet. He continues to be easily upset or excited. He may have to remain on the Feingold diet for a longer period of time or his mother may have to check his diet records for the twelve hours prior to when he is upset to see if some other unsuspected food item or contact is at fault (see chapter 3).

C. B., a five-year-old white girl, had never slept through the night as an infant. By the age of two, her parents were distraught, because she was always on the move and never able to sit still. She had a very allergic face, with itchy, puffy eyes. She sneezed often and rubbed her nose upward. Her skin was very itchy. She tended to cry often and had few friends. She had a very strong reaction to a grass-pollen skin test indicating an allergy to grass.

She was placed on the one-week diet, but her mother reported that she did not seem to be much better. When foods were fed individually during the second week, none caused obvious symptoms. About a month later, the family moved from their dusty, moldy home to a new, dry house. All C. B.'s symptoms, except the puffy eyes, were improved. Her activity score fell from 12 to 5. This patient appeared to respond mainly to a more allergy-free home.

S. P., a fourteen-year-old white female, had been overactive since about the age of seven years. She also had a bloated abdomen, halitosis, a stuffy nose, and a poor disposition. Skin tests for dust, grass, and ragweed were positive. Three weeks before she began the one-week diet (appendix B3), she had started an obesity diet. Within a week after she had been on both diets, her bloated abdomen and bad breath had improved. Her activity score fell from 16 to 8. When each food, excluded in the one-week diet, was eaten again, no consistent recurrence of symptoms was noted. The conclusion was that the improvement noted was due solely to the obesity diet. On two subsequent occasions during the next year when she stopped her obesity diet, her hyperactivity, bloating, and bad breath recurred. Her activity score also rose to the original level. S. P. must now determine which of the foods excluded or limited by the obesity diet is at fault. It is probably one of her favorites, often eaten when she is not on the diet.

5 · Food for Thought

Can foods in some way be related to common social and medical problems? This chapter briefly reviews suggested evidence that some patients with socially unacceptable behavior (delinquency, acts of violence or crime), serious mental illness, obesity, alcoholism, or convulsions might be reacting in a strange and different way to commonly eaten foods.

Are parents of battered children always to blame?

When children are beaten by their parents, this is definitely not acceptable. Some parents, however, may batter because they are driven beyond the brink of normal tolerance by their child's abnormal behavior. Parents have ups and downs, and they may be able to cope well until they have a "down" at the same time their behavior problem child has a wild "up." The real problem, however, may not be parents, but the physician's inability to recognize a child's basic medical problem. The distinct possibility exists that some parents accused of battering, have not battered: The child may have misjudged distance and speed and continually hurt himself. Let me tell Jack's story.

Jack was adopted at age fourteen weeks. He cried every day, vomited frequently, and had many bowel problems during the following two months. At that time, he developed asthma. His mother thought it was due to barley, but her doctor assured her foods could not cause asthma. Jack banged his face and head on his crib, on the floor, against anything. When he was placed in a walker, he repeatedly tipped it over. He was always bumping into something, and was, as a result, constantly black and blue. At nine months of age, he fractured his skull. He banged his head vigorously on the bathtub when he was startled by the rush of water after the faucet was turned on.

At ten months, Jack was put on a soy formula. In a few minutes he was uncontrollable. His parents could not hold him. Later, it was found that the soy formula made with tapioca caused this problem, while the one made with corn did not. At eleven months Jack ate wheat in the form of a cookie for the first time. He screamed and became so active he had to be strapped in his buggy for the next two hours. Several months later, his mother realized that new foods, including corn, were now causing symptoms.

By the time he was one and a half years old, Jack would become worse during the pollen season. His mother now knew that most grains—such as wheat, rice, oats, barley, and corn—caused symptoms and that Jack was best when these were avoided. He would flip off chairs onto the floor, roll into walls, run into table legs and doors and pick things up and heave them. Citrus fruits and bacon made him much worse in a few minutes. Once, when he ate cane sugar, Jack snarled, growled, and bit off a piece of his sister's nose. Beet sugar, however, caused no difficulty. Sometimes he had to be harnessed in bed at night to protect him from himself.

An allergist advised Jack's mother to make her home more "allergy-free." He was placed on a four-day rotary diet (see chapter 3), which eliminated the foods that his mother had noted to be a problem. In a few weeks Jack was much improved. He learned to protect himself when he fell and to walk through doorways, not into doors. It was easy for his mother to pinpoint new problem foods, because he would have trouble only at a five-day interval, whenever a suspect food was eaten. He continues to be more active than usual during the pollen season, but pollen-extract therapy has helped to relieve this.

Can other battering be due to foods?

Unfortunately, battering is not confined to parents and children. Belligerent children batter other children, especially siblings. Husbands batter wives and vice versa. Unless physicians attempt to elicit detailed information concerning possible offending foods, odors, or contacts immediately prior to acts of hostility, true answers may never be found. The battering problem is far too complex a question to be unraveled simply by food or chemical sensitivities, but investigation along this line might provide a meaningful practical method of helping a few of the batterers and batterees.

Are some delinquents, children with problems?
Can some criminals be grown-up delinquents with
chronic, severe food allergies?

Hyperactive problem children can be hostile and aggressive. Some bully, destroy, and hurt without apparent concern, thought, or regret. As children, they present testy school and social problems. As they age, their behavior may become socially and legally unacceptable (Moyer 1975, Hippchen 1976).

Could foods account for sudden, unpredictable behavior
in some children and adults?

This entire problem must be approached with extreme caution so the unscrupulous do not connive to encourage those who willfully harm others.

The following patient may furnish a glimmer of insight into a previously unrecognized problem.

Matthew was first seen at the age of fifteen years because he was hyperactive and had behavior and learning problems. For eight years, he had received Ritalin. He had year-round nasal stuffiness which was worse during the pollen season. He had had muscle and joint pains, and frequent headaches since the age of four. He was placed on the one-week diet (see appendix B3) and found to improve to such a large degree in four days, that his mother said it was "a miracle." She said the original child "had moved out." Matthew's nose, however, continued to be stuffy. When foods were re-added to his diet, his mother found he became markedly hyperactive from sugar, corn, and dyes. Repeated checks at five-day intervals confirmed that his behavior and activity changed when he ate these food items. Corn challenges repeatedly caused hyperactivity in a short while, whereas checks for sugar at five-day intervals showed this food consistently did not cause a reaction for about twelve hours. Alka-Seltzer Antacid Formula without Aspirin was said to help relieve corn-induced symptoms within twenty minutes.

Matthew was asked to swallow a series of identical capsules, some filled with sugar, others with corn, and others with control-food items to which he was not sensitive. He reacted within one and a half hours only to the corn-filled capsules.

A few weeks after he was initially tested, Matthew was caught by police while he was committing petty theft. His tearful mother explained how ashamed she was and how he could not explain his actions. As an afterthought, she mentioned that he acted oddly and looked strange at the police station. On checking his diet, we found, on that day, he had an early breakfast and then he did not eat for seven hours. Approximately one hour prior to the theft incident, he'd eaten two chocolate bars and four large peanut butter cups.

An attempt was made to duplicate the occurrences on the day when he broke the law. On the subsequent two Saturdays, he ate the identical breakfast and nothing more for seven hours. He then ate the exact same types of candy bars. On the first occasion, after forty-five minutes his nose became stuffy, his eyes glassy, and his behavior irritable and belligerent. He developed circles under his eyes. He was sent to his room. When his mother checked in a half hour she found her fifteen-year-old son acting strangely: He was eating toothpaste. On the next Saturday, he acted "like an animal" one hour after he ate the candy. He banged his head, arms, and feet against the walls of the bedroom. He talked and acted unusual for the entire rest of the day. His mother says he acted drunk. Her other children said he acted "crazy." He developed dark eye circles and "glassy" eyes. The candy contained corn, sugar, dyes, and peanuts. We subsequently checked his reaction to peanuts by allergy skin testing and found this also appeared to cause him to act and look strangely.

There is no doubt some of the effects of the challenges could have been purposeful, but the eye circles, the glassy look of his eyes and the nasal stuffiness Matthew experienced make one wonder if truly scientific studies should not be carried out concerning possible positive ways to help some persons who appear strange while breaking the law.

In my studies (Rapp 1978b, c) on the effect of diet upon activity, the parents of the four children I studied complained that stealing was a problem when the children were first brought to me. Their parents did not complain of it again, during the six months their children were on a diet and avoiding specific foods. The children did not steal during the subsequent three months, while they received sublingual food therapy without dietary restriction. To evaluate the effectiveness of the food-drop treatment after about nine months, food therapy was discontinued and the children were told to eat their normal diet. Three children reverted to stealing within three weeks. Most began by stealing sugar or candy and subsequently money to purchase sweets. All parents manifested surprise, because they had almost forgotten that theft was originally a problem.

Can such children grow into adults who cannot cope with the rules of our society?

We simply don't know (Yaryura-Tobias and Neziroglu 1975, Moyer 1975). In a book entitled *Born to Raise Hell*, Dr. Marvin Ziporyn states that Richard Speck, who was convicted of killing eight student nurses, was a compulsive sugar and candy-bar eater. Dr. Ziporyn wondered if hypoglycemia was a factor related to his emotional and uncontrollable behavior. Could corn, sugar, or chocolate be unsuspected factors?

Dr. K. E. Moyer, professor of psychology at Carnegie-Mellon University in Pittsburgh, in his recent book *Psychobiology of Aggression* (1976) reviews the role of allergy in behavior abnormalities, ranging from irritability to psychotic aggression. He infers, from his research, that hivelike swelling or edema of the brain may stimulate some nerve pathways while dulling others, causing a multiplicity of behavior patterns in affected patients.

Dr. Leonard J. Hippchen, an associate professor at Virginia Commonwealth University, suggests that biochemical deficiencies or imbalance or brain toxicity may provide answers for some hyperactive learning-disabled children who subsequently go on to delinquency or criminal behavior. In his recent book, *The Ecologic-Biochemical Approaches to Treatment of Delinquents*, he stresses the need for biochemical research not only to help prevent crime and delinquency, but to help rehabilitate criminal offenders in our society.

Can some psychiatric patients have food problems?

Dr. Theron Randolph (1962), as well as a number of ecologists and psychiatrists (Weiss and Kaufman 1971, Singh and Kay 1976, Finn and Cohen 1978), have worked in this area for several years. Some, such as Drs. Abram Hoffer and Humphrey Osmond of Canada (1978), claimed permanent remission of 80 percent of their patients who adhered to the use of large doses of vitamins C, E, and

B-complex, plus minerals. Others, such as Drs. Dohan and Grasberger (1973), found that schizophrenics who were assigned cereal-grain- or milk-free diets while in locked wards were discharged twice as rapidly as those patients fed high-cereal diets. Dr. William Philpott, in Oklahoma City (1977), and Dr. Marshall Mandell, in Boston (1977), claimed that diet and subsequent single-food challenges will relieve and precipitate symptoms in some psychiatric patients.

Dr. Richard Mackarness, a British psychiatrist, in his book *Eating Dangerously* describes how "hopeless" patients have been helped by food elimination. He discusses in detail, a twenty-eight-year-old woman named Joanna whose psychiatric history dated from the age of twenty-one. In spite of thirteen prolonged hospital admissions for psychiatric help, psychotropic drugs, and electroshock therapy, a panel of psychiatrists decided a lobotomy was necessary. Dr. Mackarness asked if he might investigate the possibility of a food sensitivity and was granted time to investigate this prior to neurosurgery. After being given only bottled water for five days, Joanna was acting and talking normally. Individual food challenges confirmed that wheat, among other foods, caused her to act in a hostile and abnormal manner. Double-blind challenges confirmed that certain food items repeatedly caused abnormal behavior. Joanna remains well, as long as she adheres to her diet. Neurosurgery was not necessary.

Could alcoholism be related to food problems?

Dr. Theron Randolph has been applying the principles of ecology to study alcoholism for over thirty years. His major contribution in this area (Randolph 1950, 1976b) included the following observations. Alcoholics are most often corn or wheat sensitive. Additional ingredients in liquor, which cause symptoms, are other grains (malt), grapes, yeast, flavorings, and sugars of various types. Most people can drink or not drink but this is not true for alcoholics. Some highly food-allergic persons can become alcoholics the first time they take a drink. Patients who appear drunk after one or two drinks or who have extreme hangovers from a small amount of alcohol are often found to have a sensitivity to an ingredient commonly found in their regular diet, as well as in their favorite liquor. Dr. Randolph questioned forty-five members of Alcoholics Anonymous. He found all but one had a definite, positive history of allergy. He believes that alcohol is so rapidly absorbed that addiction in allergic persons is not infrequent. Alcoholics feel better when they drink because imbibing not only gives them a lift, it also prevents withdrawal symptoms. Thus the vicious cycle develops. Dr. Randolph and other ecologists have found that four- or five-day hospital fasts may break the cycle and allow the patient to lose his intense need for alcohol. It is interesting that after an alcoholic has fasted four days, if wheat is the cause of his symptoms, the ingestion of a small quantity of wheat can produce complaints identical to those noted after a bout of drinking (Randolph 1976b, Frazier 1974, Breneman 1978).

Is obesity related to an allergic food addiction problem?

Some ecologists believe that, like some alcoholics, some obese persons may have a food addiction for sugars and carbohydrates. They also suffer from withdrawal symptoms if they try not to eat, so they persist in eating. Dr. Richard Mackarness initially investigated various diets to help obesity and was surprised to find that his diets also relieved multiple chronic allergic symptoms (1976). More scientific study is needed to investigate these problems in an unprejudiced manner.

What other problems might be related to food allergies?

Anorexia Nervosa.   Could the ingestion of certain foods cause a patient to lose the desire to eat?

Infertility.   Could foods cause the oviducts to go into spasm, similar to an asthmatic's bronchi?

Nymphomania or Impotence.   Could foods alter one's sex drive or ability? It has been observed that some females manifest extremely exaggerated sexual interest only when they eat certain foods premenstrually. Could some men also have food-related sexual problems?

Speech Problems.   Could stuttering, rapid, high-pitched, or unclear speech be related to foods. Parents of hyperactive children often comment that their child's speech changes when they eat foods to which they are sensitive.

Seizures.   There are reports of altered brainwaves noted in association with the ingestion of certain foods (Speer 1970, Davison 1949, 1952). Dr. Richard Mackarness (1976) confirmed the role of foods in this problem during a recent British television demonstration. He placed a few drops of liquified instant coffee

under a young woman's tongue and showed this made her convulse
in a few minutes. Dr. Theron Randolph has noted that odors, as
well as foods, can cause similar symptoms.

Solid scientific evidence is beginning to be published which
indicates that some nephrosis, arthritis, and blood vessel and
cardiac problems can be caused by food and/or chemical sensitivities (Rea 1976, 1977, 1978, Sandberg et al. 1977).

Suicides. A number of depressed, teenage children in my
practice have admitted that they tried to commit suicide because
they were depressed, unhappy, and not improving. Solving their
food problem appears to have relieved their multiple symptoms
and restored their hope and confidence.

Could mental retardation be related to food allergies?

There is a long-term detailed report in medical literature by an
allergist, a neurologist, and a psychologist concerning eight
children who had learning disabilities, hyperactivity, fatigue, and
incoordination (Millman et al. 1976). They were treated with a
combination of diet and allergy-injection therapy for dust, molds,
and pollens. All children showed marked improvement in their
temperament, disposition, and ability to learn after treatment. As
their physical symptoms subsided, their psychological functioning
also improved. Their neurological symptoms did not change
during the twelve months of study. Their IQ's rose by 10 to 25
points. Of this group only one child was a dull normal, but all the
children were poor achievers in school.

In 1978, I performed a small research study on a group of eleven
hyperactive learning-disabled children. Three children of this
group had mental retardation. It was found that these three
children appeared to respond favorably to a preservative-free diet
and some also responded to sublingual food therapy. The foods
treated included milk, wheat, eggs, cocoa, sugar, corn, artificial
food coloring, tomatoes, peanuts, grapes, apples, and oranges. One
youngster was observed by the speech therapist to speak more
clearly and slowly, to be more alert and cooperative, and to
concentrate and anticipate much better than she had ever been
able to do in the past. In addition, her parents noted that she was
less restless, had fewer emotional outbursts, and became less angry.
Her skin became less scaly and her nose and intestinal symptoms
subsided. When the study was completed, she was allowed, once

again, to eat preservatives, and, at the same time food therapy was discontinued. The change was dramatic: all of her original symptoms recurred within ten days. When preservatives were eliminated from her diet again, she became less agitated and argumentative. Her other symptoms, however, did not subside until she resumed food therapy. Further long-term studies are planned to monitor her IQ and her ability to learn and communicate.

A second retarded youngster in this group was a thirteen-year-old boy who had wet his bed almost nightly since infancy. During the six weeks when he was on a preservative-free diet, this problem gradually improved, so that he was wetting only one night out of seven. Within a week of resuming the ingestion of preservative-containing foods, he began to wet again every night, and when preservatives were discontinued, two weeks later, his symptoms again improved dramatically.

During the three-week period when he received food therapy in addition to the preservative-free diet, his teacher noted dramatic improvement in the child's schoolwork, which had not been evident earlier while he was receiving placebo food treatment for three weeks. His teacher stated the boy "talked less, had a longer attention span, needed less individual attention, asked fewer questions, seemed less confused, and could concentrate better."

The third youngster in the study, a fifteen-year-old boy, ate a preservative-free diet. His disposition, activity, behavior, and ability to concentrate all improved. Food therapy did not seem to alter his symptoms. When the diet was discontinued, his symptoms flared again and, in addition, he began to soil his underwear with bowel movements. When he was again placed on a preservative-free diet the boy's symptoms subsided. Further studies are presently being conducted on this youngster.

This small study, in itself, only suggests that children with retardation can be helped if their allergies are treated. Larger, long-term, well-controlled and designed studies concerning the role of diet in retarded children appears to be a sensible endeavor. This is particularly true if the mentally deficient youngsters also have evidence of possible allergy as detailed in chapter 3. An attempt should be made in such children to note if there is any improvement associated with making their homes more allergy-free (appendix E1), placing them on an allergy-free diet (appendix B3), or treating them with injection therapy for pollen, dust, etc.

In 1978, Dr. Dan O'Banion and his associates in Denton, Texas, conducted a special thirty-one-day study on an eight-year-old autistic child, using a dietary approach. After an appropriate baseline period of observation, the child was placed on a diet. He was then fed individual food items while various parameters were carefully monitored—activity, amount of laughter, and such disruptive behavior as screaming, scratching, biting and throwing objects. Wheat, oats, tomatoes, sugar, and dairy products were found to be major offending items. Some foods were found to cause immediate reactions which lasted only a short while, but other foods repeatedly caused delayed-onset reactions which could persist as long as three days.

In 1979, Simeon and associates helped 6 of 8 autistic children using Cromolyn before meals. This drug relieves allergy and the favorable response in these children indicates foods may be related to some autism.

Is treatment for food and chemical sensitivities a panacea for many social ills?

Of course not. Many complex variables contribute to our social problems, and there certainly is no one, single, simple answer. We must, however, realize that foods and chemicals do adversely affect some children and adults, contributing directly or indirectly to unacceptable or antisocial behavior. By recognizing such a possibility, perhaps we can help this select subpopulation significantly.

Should parents attempt to alter the school lunch program?

In many communities parents are presently organizing in an effort to alter the types of foods served in schools. The luncheons frequently contain high-caloric, carbohydrate foods such as pastries, cakes, cookies, spaghetti, noodles, pizza, and sweet items. It has been suggested that school lunches should be free of additives, preservatives, artificial coloring, sugar, and other food items which so frequently appear to be associated with hyperactivity, behavior, and learning problems. It also has been questioned whether vending machines in schools should dispense snacks consisting of carbonated, artificially colored and flavored beverages, candies of various types, and corn or potato chip snacks which contain additives and preservatives. Will hungry children eat fresh fruits if these are available? I believe definitive answers cannot be given at this time. Evidence is slowly accumulating that behavior and learning are indeed affected by foods. If more confirmation appears during the next few years, parents may be able to insist that nutritious food items be given to their children at school. Some small schools, in particular, presently serve excellent homemade food to children, but there is a marked variation in the menus served within communities and in different areas of the country.

What could cause so many food-related problems?

When one ponders food sensitivities, the major perplexing question is, why do so many children and adults appear to have problems from so many foods? It does not seem natural or right. Is there some other basic deficiency which causes the body to malfunction? What causes such a deficiency? Is there some chemical, enzyme, vitamin, mineral, trace metal, or unknown which could be given to normalize a body so food could be eaten without difficulty?

Could our bodies be in a delicate balance which tolerates a limited, but fairly wide range of deviation from normal? When the combination of environmental contamination and life stresses are too great, do the stabilizing mechanisms falter completely? Is this why so many youngsters presently appear to be afflicted with hyperactivity? Is this why an inordinate number of normally non-offending foods and odors suddenly appear to cause difficulty in previously well adults? Again, we don't have the answers, but many patients with complex food and chemical allergies date the onset of their problems to a serious accident, infection, emotional upset, or hormonal change. We cannot be sure that such relationships are not pure coincidence rather than cause and effect, but if they are valid, they do indeed give us food for thought.

It will be years before we have answers, but the ultimate solution to food problems is not a drug to mask symptoms, a diet which omits offending foods or sublingual or injection food therapy. We must determine how to restabilize the body so foods do not cause medical problems. As Dr. Joe Nichols suggests in *Please, Doctor, Do Something*, we must correct our diet so our foods and beverages do not harm our bodies. We must urge the government and legislators to realign their priorities and provide meaningful protection. Must our health be compromised because of powerful lobbies? In return for economic prosperity and modern methods, can we continue to allow subtle and overt, ever-increasing food, water, and air contamination?

Appendices

Appendix A · Additional Patient Reports

A1: Scott

This white male youngster was eleven years old when first seen in my office. As an infant he was very active. Scott broke his leg after he learned to walk because he charged into walls and furniture. Many other members in his family had allergies. He was in a special class for children with learning disabilities. He had had slight nose symptoms throughout the year for several years. He had occasional abdominal pain. Gas was a problem after eating, almost every day, since he was very young. He tended to have leg cramps at bedtime. He sucked his lower lip. His behavior was unpredictable and bad. He was irritable, grouchy, clumsy, restless, hostile, and talked and cried too much. He fought with his brother and schoolmates, and had no friends. On one day, his mother received nineteen calls from neighbors because of his behavior. He was sassy and tended to rave on and on in a senseless manner. At times he almost acted "insane." He had many school problems because of his lack of discipline and easy distractibility. He was not affectionate. He had been seen by a neurologist and psychologist for therapy sessions for six months without obvious help.

He was placed on the diet which omitted all milk, wheat, eggs, cocoa, corn, sugar and dyes (see appendix B3). Within a day, his leg cramps were gone and in two days his activity was better. His mother said by the end of the week her "bananas kid was gone." He was having only one fight a day whereas before he had had many. He was able to play with the neighborhood children for the first time in his life. He talked less. He even "took a nap."

He was quiet. He became loving and kissed his parents. He no longer had belly gas and stopped sucking his lower lip. He didn't cry all the time. Church previously had been a hassle; now he was quiet during the entire service.

Two teachers called his mother to comment on his marked improvement in school. His activity score, after the one-week diet, fell from 19 to 1 and fourteen weeks later, the score was 0. Six months later his score was only 2. His mother was delighted that he had changed so much. She found he had a nice personality, which had previously been completely hidden.

Scott's skin test for allergy to dust and pollen showed no sensitivity. When individual foods were re-added to his diet, he reacted to sugar and dyes. Foods with a little red, yellow, or blue dye caused him to rave and become irritable and made his legs ache. This reaction occurred within a few minutes and lasted at least a day. After drinking colored beverages, his teacher called to state he was argumentative, threw things, and did not listen. He could eat a little sugar, but if he ate too much he had a delayed reaction. Usually in two to four hours, he became argumentative and disagreeable, as well as hyperactive. Alka-Seltzer Antacid Formula without Aspirin helped these symptoms. He was eventually allowed to eat the foods to which he was sensitive, and had no difficulty if he used appropriate food-drop therapy under his tongue each day (see chapter 4).

A2: **Matthew**

Matthew, a twelve-year-old Puerto Rican male, was hyperactive, but he was not on drugs to control his activity. He'd been overactive since infancy. For the first two years of his life, he slept only three hours a night and napped only two hours a day. He was known to have pollen and dust allergies and had been well treated with extract therapy for five years.

His mother described this as a typical day: "In the morning Matthew was stuffy and tired. He was cranky and would get upset over homework not done, cry, call himself stupid, and pester his sister. When he arrived home from school, he immediately took off shoes and did somersaults through the house. He thumped and jumped about the house, or would lie and watch television with his hands and feet tapping and banging away constantly. At dinner he rapped his fork and knife on the plate, picked up and handled things on the table, turned the salt shaker upside down, kicked the table and his sister, and, intermittently, throughout the meal, jumped up to do somersaults in the living room. After supper he would try to do his homework. He would get upset because he forgot some books and say he was stupid. He'd write two or three words, rip up the sheet because of an error and do this about five to six times. He'd cry, get upset again, and the next morning either lose or forget his homework. At bedtime he would say that his muscles and belly had ached all day (a problem since his early years), and it would take an hour and a half to get to sleep. He said his mind was speeding and he could not relax. He'd roll and toss all night with bad dreams and talking. During the day he talked constantly about anything and would not listen. He never ate more than half a meal, never had an appetite. His nose was usually stuffy."

After four days on the multiple food allergy diet (appendix B3) Matthew was obviously much better and by seven days, he had markedly improved. His mother reported he was less active, less easily aggravated, friendlier, happier, and had lost all his aches and his cough. His appetite was much better.

When foods were re-added, it was found that milk caused depression, irritability, and excess talking. Chocolate caused his nose to run and bellyaches, but did not affect his activity. Corn caused light-headedness, bellyaches, excess talking, and inability to sleep. Red dyes caused irritability, he seemed "spaced out." He'd forget what he was saying and develop nose stuffiness and irritability. Eggs and sugar caused no symptoms.

To prove his milk sensitivity, he was given unmarked capsules, some containing milk and others containing sugar. He became depressed and developed a bellyache from milk-filled capsules, while the sugar-filled capsules had no effect.

In time, his mother also observed that chlorinated water caused a bellyache and soy oil or foods packed in this oil, such as tuna fish (but not soybeans) caused irritability and muscle aches. Wheat made him very hyperactive, irritable, and depressed.

His mother rechecked his wheat sensitivity at a five-day interval by feeding him wheat crackers at 10 A.M. after he had avoided wheat for four full days. "He argued with his sister and was sent to his room by 10:45 A.M. He didn't care. He was listless and fidgety for a while. He became hyperactive. He took paper and made a fire on the basement floor. He turned a hose on it, sprayed the floor, then ran and slid and played in the water. He was giddy all day, aware of the happy feeling and said it sure beat being depressed. During dinner he threw down his fork and started doing cartwheels. He became more reasonable by 9:30 P.M., but was still hyperactive."

His activity score one week after the diet was begun had fallen from 18 to 1, and three and five months later, while continuing to avoid milk, chocolate, corn, wheat, and food coloring, the score was still 1. His teacher commented that Matthew was better in school, and after four weeks on the diet, his grades had definitely improved. He now relaxes, watches TV without wiggling, eats well, sleeps quietly, awakens refreshed and happy.

He began under-the-tongue food-drop treatment after about five months of avoiding his problem foods (see chapter 4). He found that he could then eat most foods that previously had caused symptoms in moderation without difficulty. His activity score was 0 after three months of food treatment. When he was given his food-treatment drops in a double-blind manner, he could distinguish the one bottle of real drops from the two bottles that contained a solution which tasted and looked the same, but did not contain foods.

His mother placed his sister on the same diet while she was checking Matthew and found that a little milk caused her to become nasty, depressed, and so unhappy she cried for hours. She improved remarkably on a milk-free diet.

Eighteen months later, both children continue to be markedly improved, but their diets must be watched carefully. An excessive amount of some foods continues to cause symptoms in spite of treatment. Chemical allergies continue to be a problem because avoidance is difficult.

Appendix B · Diets and Diet Aids

B1: **Food and Allergy and Other Related Problems**

FOODS WHICH OFTEN CAUSE ALLERGY

Milk	Potato
Corn	Beef
Wheat	Onions
Eggs	Soy
Chocolate	Peas
Sugar (beet, corn, or cane)	Peanuts
Food coloring	Berries
Tomatoes	Fish
Citrus	Chicken
Cinnamon	Yeast
Coffee (in adults)	Pork
Alcohol (in adults)	

RELATED AND UNRELATED FOODS

A sensitivity to one of these is related to the others in same group. If one bothers you, the others also may be a problem.

Apple and pear	Peach, plum, cherry, apricot, almond
Avocado and cinnamon	
Beet and spinach	Peanut, pea, bean, licorice
Carrot, celery, and parsley	Onion, garlic, asparagus, chives
Chocolate and cola drinks	Orange, grapefruit, lemon, lime
Cranberry and blueberry	Shrimp, lobster, crab
Cucumber and melons	Walnut and pecan
Dates and coconut	Wheat, corn, rye

Used by permission of Syntex Laboratories. From the booklet *Food Sensitivity Diets.* © 1978 by Doris J. Rapp.

UNRELATED FOODS

A sensitivity to one of the following items is in *no way related* to any other listed item.

Almond and any other nut	Peanut and any other nut
Black and red pepper	Raisin (grape) and prune (plum)
Clove, ginger, cinnamon	Tuna and shrimp
Coffee and tea	Wheat and buckwheat
Crab and clam	White potato and sweet potato

MEDICAL PROBLEMS AND POSSIBLE MAJOR FOOD OR OTHER SUSPECTS

Hives. Chocolate, milk, eggs, peanuts, cinnamon, preservatives, and artificial coloring or flavoring. Seasonal strawberries, melons or tomato. Aspirin, penicillin, other antibiotics.

Eczema. Milk, chocolate, nuts, peanuts, egg. Mold spores, yeast, dust and pollen.

Nose Problems. Milk, orange, corn, chocolate, wheat, artificial food coloring, egg.

Ear Problems. Milk, eggs, chocolate, peanut, corn, chicken, wheat. Dust, pets, molds.

Wheezing or Asthma. Milk, eggs, wheat or any grain, fish or shellfish, peanuts, cocoa, corn, nuts, wheat, onion, garlic. Aspirin, tartrazine dyes.

Allergic-Tension-Fatigue Syndrome (hyperactivity, fatigue, hostility, irritability, emotional lability, depression, speech problems). Artificial coloring, preservatives, sugar (cane or beet), milk, corn, cocoa, wheat, eggs, oranges, apples, grapes, peanuts, tomatoes, and food additives or artificial flavorings. Dust, mold spores, and pollen. Odors from perfume or chemicals.

Convulsions. Milk, yeast (vitamin B) chicken, or any other food.

Ulcers in Mouth. Citrus, pickles, apples, coffee, chocolate, potatoes, nuts and cinnamon.

Colitis. Milk, wheat, eggs, corn, cocoa, nuts, orange, pork, beef, chicken, peanut, sugar.

Gall Bladder Disease. Eggs, pork, onion, chicken, milk, coffee, oranges, corn, beans, nuts.

Ulcer (Duodenal). Milk, chicken, wheat, corn, eggs, beef, tomatoes, coffee, tea, oranges, avocadoes, peach, potatoes, barley, chocolate, grapes, peanuts, and spices.

Bladder Problems (Bed-wetting, Frequent or Urgent Wetting). Milk, eggs, citrus, corn, wheat, pork, tomato, chicken, cola, cocoa, onion, fish, cinnamon, apple, peanuts, preservatives and artificial colors. Oranges are the most common food causing adult cystitis. Molds.

MEDICAL PROBLEMS (CONT)

Kidney Problems (such as nephrosis). Milk, wheat.

High Blood Pressure and Irregular Heart Beat, Blood Vessel Problems. Chocolate, corn, nut, pork, peanuts, coffee, milk wheat, rice, beef, shrimp, seafood, chicken, apples, peanut butter. Chemical odors, such as natural gas fumes, gasoline fumes, chlorine, air pollution, auto exhaust, soft plastic, cleaning chemicals (Lysol-phenol), perfume, polyurethane, tobacco smoke, polyester fabrics, fiberglass, Naugahyde, new carpeting, formaldehyde, pesticides, pest strips, and foam rubber.

Headache. Milk, chocolate, chicken, coffee, egg, corn, peanut, peas, beans, cinnamon, pork, garlic, and food coloring. Pollen, mold spores, dust, pets, air pollution, auto exhaust, tobacco smoke, paint fumes, perfumes, chemical odors, natural gas.

Arthritis, Joint Pain, or Rheumatism. Pork (bacon, ham), lard, milk, chicken, chocolate, wheat, beef, coffee, eggs, and artificial food coloring.

Recurrent Infection. Milk, eggs, corn, wheat, cinnamon, or other spices, citrus (oranges, lemons, limes, grapefruits), chocolate, cola.

Fluid Retention. Pork.

B2: **Diet Record Sheets**

FIRST WEEK FOOD DIARY   **When foods are omitted from diet**

Record EVERYTHING eaten (gum, medications, etc.) each day.

	Day 1	Day 2	Day 3
Breakfast			
Snacks			
Lunch			
Snacks			
Dinner			
Snacks			
Comment			

Used by permission of Syntex Laboratories. From the booklet *Food Sensitivity Diets*.
© 1978 by Doris J. Rapp.

Record in RED when any symptom begins each day.

Day 4	Day 5	Day 6	Day 7

SECOND WEEK FOOD DIARY   When foods are to be re-added

Record EVERYTHING eaten (gum, medications, etc.) each day

	Day 1	Day 2	Day 3
	Excess milk, dairy products, cottage cheese all day.	Excess bread and wheat cereal all day. (No preservatives)	Excess sugar all day. Sugar cubes.
Breakfast			
Snacks			
Lunch			
Snacks			
Dinner			
Snacks			
Comment			

Record in RED when any symptom begins each day.

Day 4	Day 5	Day 6	Day 7
Excess eggs all day. If eggs disliked give in foods.	Excess cocoa or chocolate all day.	Excess dyed foods all day. Jell-O, fruited drinks, candy.	Excess corn all day. Popcorn, whole kernel and corn flakes.

B3: **One-Week Multiple Food Allergy Diet**

The one-week diet and those in appendixes B5 through B11 are all used in conjunction with the record sheets in B2 as part of the diet plan to help patients whose hyperactivity may be due to their diet. "How to Do the Diet" in chapter 4 provides a detailed discussion of how these diet sheets are to be used. Consult this chapter before trying any part of the diet plan. Do not use the diet unless your physician has been consulted and approved it. Do not do it if the patient has either asthma or severe food allergy.

For one full week, this diet omits all milk and dairy products, wheat (bread, cake, baked goods), eggs, nuts, sugar, chocolate (cola), corn, citrus, preservatives and dyes. It allows meats, fruits, and most vegetables (no peas or corn). If symptoms are not improved after one week, a second week may be tried, but if symptoms are still not improved, then there is no need to proceed further with the diet since it is unlikely that any of the foods omitted during the diet-week are factors related to the symptoms.

On the one-week diet, only the *allowed* foods may be selected, combined, and eaten in any quantity, for any meal. No other food items should be eaten or used in preparation or in cooking. If an item is not listed, it should not be eaten. If one of the allowed foods causes obvious severe or serious allergy, do not include it in your individual diet. Foods with an (*) must be prepared exactly as suggested in appendix B4.

Juices marked with an (**) contain no sugar, artificial color, or preservatives. Juices marked with an (***) may contain corn and sugar without being so marked. You can make any fruit into fresh juice by mixing it with water in the blender; if necessary it can be sweetened with pure honey or pure maple syrup.

ALLOWED

Cereals
Rice—Rice Puffs only
Oats—Oatmeal made with honey
Barley

Fruits
Any fresh fruit, except citrus
Canned (if in their own juice
    without artificial color, sugar, or
    preservatives)

FORBIDDEN

Cereals
Foods containing wheat flour
Corn

Fruits
Fresh frozen or canned***
Citrus (orange, lemon, lime,
    grapefruit)

Used by permission of Syntex Laboratories. From the booklet *Food Sensitivity Diets.* ©1978 by Doris J. Rapp.

ALLOWED

Vegetables
Any *fresh* vegetable
French fries (homemade)
Potatoes

Meats
Chicken or turkey (non-basted)
Veal or beef
Pork
Lamb
Fish, tuna, lobster

Beverages
Tea with honey
Water
Grape juice—bottled**(Welch's)
Frozen apple juice**(Lincoln's)
Diet colorless cream soda
Pure pineapple juice

Snacks
Potato chips (no additives)
Ry-Krisp crackers and pure honey
Raisins (unsulphured)

Miscellaneous
Pure honey
Homemade vinegar and oil
   dressing
Sea salt
Pepper
Saccharin or artificial sweetener
Homemade soups

FORBIDDEN

Vegetables
Fresh frozen or canned***
Corn
Mixed vegetables
Peas

Meats
Luncheon meats, wieners
Bacon
Artificially colored hamburger or
   meat
Ham
Dyed salmon
Breaded meats
Meats with stuffing

Beverages
Milk or any type of dairy products
   (cheese, yogurt)
Fruit beverages except those so
   specified
Kool-Aid
Coffee Rich (yellow dye)
7-Up, Squirt, Teem, Cola, Dr. Pepper

Snacks
Corn chips—Fritos
Chocolate or anything with cocoa
Hard candy
Ice cream or sherbet

Miscellaneous
Sugar
Bread, (rye, potato), cake, cookies except
   on special recipes
Eggs
Dyed (colored) vitamins, pills,
   mouth wash, toothpaste,
   medicines, cough syrups, etc.
Jelly or jam
Jell-O
Margarine or diet spreads (dyes and
   corn)
Peanut butter
Sorbitol (corn)
Nuts

SUGGESTIONS

Breakfast
Dry cereal or put allowed juices or
   honey water on it
Fruit
Meat
Salad—vegetables or fruit
Potato chips

Lunch
Vegetable salad
Fresh fruit or fruit salad
Drumstick or chicken slices
Chicken on Ry-Krisp crackers
Pork chops (not breaded)
Apple crisp*
Homemade soup

SUMMARY LIST OF ALLOWED FOODS

Cereals or Grains
Oatmeal
Barley
Rice
Ry-Krisp, nonseasoned (grind for
   cereal)
Fearn Rice Baking Mix (waffles,
   pancakes)

Vegetables (fresh only)
Cabbage:
   Cole slaw*
Carrots
White potato
   Mashed
   Fried
   Boiled
   Baked
   French fries (homemade)
   Chips (no additives)
   Salad*
   Flour
Sweet potato
   Baked
   Candied*
Green beans
Tomatoes
   Raw
Lettuce

Spinach
Celery
Green pepper
Broccoli
Cucumbers
Beets
Asparagus
Onions
Brussels sprouts
Baked squash
Chives
Tossed salad with French dressing*
Spanish rice*
Waldorf salad*

Beverages
Soybean milk (drugstore or chain
   store) Neo Mull Soy, Nursoy,
   Isomil
Juice or carbonated beverages (only
   if without sugar or dyes)
   grape
   apple
   peach or apricot nectar
   pineapple
   pear
   cranberry (without corn syrup)
   tea
   black coffee
Some of these can be used on cereal

ALLOWED FOODS (CONT)

Desserts
Carob brownies*
Apple crisp*
Tapioca—fruit juice

Meats
Beef
   pot roast
   stew*
   swiss steak*
   liver
   meat loaf*
Chicken (not breaded)
   baked
   salad*
Turkey
Fish
   tuna
   other
Pork
   chops (not breaded)
   roast
Lamb
Hash*

Condiments
Sea salt
Pepper
Ginger
Cinnamon
Vinegar
   cider
   white

Paprika
Bayleaf
Thyme
Sucaryl
Saccharin
Maple syrup (pure) or sugar
Honey (pure)
Date sugar

Fruits (fresh only)
Bananas
Apples
   raw
   baked
   sauce
Grapes
   raisins (unsulphured, health food
   store)
Peaches
Pears
Pineapple

Miscellaneous
Egg-free baking powder (obtain
   at health food store)
Water
Vegetable (not corn)
   cooking oil (safflower)
Mayonnaise*
Potato flour
Potato meal
Willow Run Margarine
Crisco

B4: **Recipes for the One-Week Multiple Food Allergy Diet**

MEATS

Special Hash

1 green pepper, diced, fresh
3 medium onions, diced, fresh
3 tablespoons Crisco
1½ pounds ground beef
1 fresh tomato

¾ cup water
1½ teaspoons salt
¼ teaspoon pepper
3 cups chopped, cooked potatoes
(about 4)

Saute green pepper, and onions in Crisco in a large skillet until onions are transparent. Add meat and continue to cook until lightly browned. Combine tomato, water, and seasonings, and add to meat mixture. Then add potatoes and cook until liquid is nearly evaporated, about 15 minutes, turning occasionally. *Makes 4 hearty servings.*

Special Baked Chicken

Chicken parts
¼ cup oil or melted Crisco

1 cup finely crushed potato chips
(no preservatives)
Salt and pepper

Preheat oven to 400 degrees. Dip chicken in oil. Drain. Sprinkle with salt and pepper and roll in crushed chips. Arrange in greased, shallow baking dish. Cover tightly with foil. Bake 45 minutes until tender. Uncover for at least 15 minutes to brown chicken.

Beef Stew

1 pound beef, cut in 1-inch cubes
2 tablespoons safflower oil or
     melted Crisco
¼ cup chopped onion
3 cups boiling water
1 tablespoon salt
⅛ teaspoon pepper

1 small bay leaf
Dash of thyme
¾ cup diced carrots, fresh
¾ cup diced potatoes
8 to 10 small white onions, fresh
1 cup boiling water
5 tablespoons potato starch

Brown beef in fat in a large saucepan. Add onion and saute until golden brown. Add 3 cups boiling water and seasonings, cover and simmer 1½ to 2 hours, or until meat is nearly tender. Add vegetables and continue cooking for 30 minutes longer, or until vegetables are done. Add 1 cup

Used by permission of Syntex Laboratories. From the booklet *Food Sensitivity Diets.*
© 1978 by Doris J. Rapp.

boiling water. Add a few tablespoons cold water to potato starch and mix to a paste. Add to stew. Cook and stir until slightly thickened. *Serves 3.*

Special Meat Loaf

2 pounds ground beef	1½ teaspoons salt
⅓ cups Minute Tapioca	¼ teaspoon pepper
⅓ cup onion, finely chopped	1½ cups fresh tomatoes, peeled, mashed

Combine all ingredients, mixing well. Then pack into a 9″ × 5″ × 3″ loaf pan. Bake at 350 degrees for 1 to 1¼ hours. Unmold on serving platter and slice. May be served hot or cold. *Makes 6 to 8 servings.*

Swiss Steak

1 pound round steak	Chopped onion and celery
Potato meal	½ cup water
Sea salt and pepper	1½ cup peeled tomatoes, fresh or
3 tablespoons safflower oil or melted Crisco	home canned

Dredge the steak well in potato meal seasoned with salt and pepper. Brown meat in melted fat. Add remaining ingredients. Cover and bake at 325 degrees for 1½ hours. *Makes 2 to 3 servings.*

VEGETABLES

Oven-Browned Potatoes

Pare medium-sized potatoes and boil for 10 minutes. Place the parboiled potatoes around the roast in a roasting pan an hour or more before the meat is to be served. Turn the potatoes once or twice while they are roasting. If the potatoes do not brown sufficiently in the oven, they may be removed to a separate pan and placed under the broiler for a few minutes before serving. Browned potatoes may also be cooked in a separate pan with meat fat or safflower oil. Allow plenty of space between the potatoes so that they will brown, and roast at 375 degrees for about 1 hour. *Makes 4 servings.*

Candied Sweet Potatoes

4 medium sweet potatoes	2 tablespoons Crisco or safflower
1 cup honey	oil

Peel the potatoes and cut in half lengthwise. Arrange in a baking dish. Mix the remaining ingredients and pour over the potatoes. Bake at 375 degrees for 50 minutes. *Makes 4 servings.*

Spanish Rice

¼ cup safflower oil or Crisco
1 medium onion, thinly sliced
½ medium green pepper, diced
1⅓ cups Minute Rice

1½ cups hot water
2 eight-ounce cans tomato sauce
   (only if homemade)
1 teaspoon sea salt
Dash of pepper

Melt fat in saucepan or skillet. Add onion, green pepper, and precooked rice. Cook and stir over high heat until slightly browned. Add remaining ingredients. Mix well. Bring quickly to a boil—reduce heat and simmer, uncovered, for 5 minutes. *Makes 4 servings.*

SALADS

Special Boiled Mayonnaise

1½ tablespoons potato starch flour
½ teaspoon sea salt
¼ teaspoon dry mustard
2 teaspoons honey
¼ cup cold water

⅔ cup boiling water
1 tablespoon white vinegar
½ cup vegetable oil (not corn)
Salt
Pepper

Combine the potato starch, salt, dry mustard, and honey in a saucepan and stir to a smooth paste with the ¼ cup of cold water. Add the boiling water and cook only until mixture is clear. Remove from heat and cool to lukewarm. Add the vinegar and oil, beating constantly. Season with salt and pepper. *Makes 1¾ cups.*

French Dressing

1 cup vegetable oil
⅓ cup apple cider vinegar
1 teaspoon sea salt
2 teaspoons pure honey

1 teaspoon paprika
⅛ teaspoon pepper
2 teaspoons water

In a jar combine all of the above ingredients. Cover tightly and shake well. *Makes 1⅓ cups.*

Cole Slaw

Shredded cabbage
Grated carrots

Minced green pepper
Special boiled mayonnaise

Mix vegetables and blend with special boiled mayonnaise.

Waldorf Salad

1 apple, cored and chopped
Celery, chopped

1 tablespoon unsulphured raisins
Special boiled mayonnaise

Combine apple, raisins, and celery. Mix lightly with special boiled mayonnaise until all pieces are coated. Chill. *Serves 2.*

Special Potato Salad

Sliced warm boiled potatoes
Chopped chives (optional), fresh
Sea salt and pepper to taste
Grated onion, fresh

1 tablespoon apple cider vinegar
Chopped celery, fresh
Special boiled mayonnaise

Combine warm potatoes, chives, salt, pepper, onion, and vinegar. Stir well and chill. Meanwhile, mix celery and boiled mayonnaise and chill. Combine potato and special boiled mayonnaise mixtures before serving. *Makes 3–4 servings.*

Chicken Salad

2 cups cooked chicken, diced
½ cup celery, chopped
¼ cup onion, grated, fresh

Sea salt and pepper to taste
Special boiled mayonnaise

Combine all ingredients and toss lightly to coat chicken with special boiled mayonnaise. *Makes 2–3 servings.*

DESSERTS

Apple Crisp

4 cups sliced cooking apples
1 tablespoon pure lemon juice
1 cup Quaker or Mother's Oats
    (quick or old-fashioned, un-
    cooked)

½ cup honey
1 teaspoon cinnamon
¼ cup melted Crisco

Place apples in shallow baking dish. Sprinkle with lemon juice. Combine remaining ingredients; mix until crumbly. Sprinkle crumb mixture over apples. Bake in preheated moderate oven (375 degrees) for 30 minutes or until apples are tender. *Makes 6 servings.*

Fruit Juice Tapioca

¼ cup Minute Tapioca
2¼ cups apple juice (pure)

¾ cup pure honey
Dash of sea salt

Mix all the ingredients in a saucepan and let stand 5 minutes. Cook and stir over medium heat until mixture comes to a boil. Cool 20 minutes. Then stir well and spoon into dessert dishes. Chill. *Makes 3 servings.*

Carob Brownies

¼ cup lima bean flour
¾ cup soy flour
1 cup rice flour
1 cup carob powder
1½ teaspoon baking powder
1 teaspoon sea salt

1 cup chopped nuts
½ cup honey
¼ cup safflower oil
1 teaspoon vanilla
1¼ cup water

Combine flours, carob powder, baking powder, salt, and nuts. Mix honey, oil, vanilla, and water. Add dry ingredients, stir well, and pour into a 8″ × 8″ × 2″ baking pan. Bake in 325-degree oven for 45 minutes to get cakelike brownies, for 35 minutes to get chewy brownies. *Makes 16 brownies.*

The following ice cream is made without milk but it *contains sugar.* Be sure a corn-free oil is used. Do not eat unless you are certain sugar is not a próblem.

Old-Fashioned Homemade Ice Cream

4 cans Isomil
2 packets (1 tablespoon/packet
    unflavored gelatin—soften in ½
    cup cold water)

1¼ cup sugar—add to gelatin and
    heat slowly to dissolve sugar
    and gelatin; cool
¼ cup safflower oil
7 teaspoons vanilla extract

Mix all ingredients and freeze in a 1-gallon or 5-quart ice cream freezer. After the mix is frozen, remove and store in freezing compartment of refrigerator. Any fruits you like which are included in your diet may be added to recipe prior to freezing after being mashed or pureed in a blender. Fruit flavors taste best.

For other soybean milk recipes write for the free *Neo-Mull-Soy® Recipe Book*:

Ross Laboratories, Inc.
    625 Cleveland Avenue
    Columbus, OH 43216

Other recipes and food tips may be found in the cook books listed in appendix C4.

B5: **Diet to Check for Milk Allergy**

If you must remove milk from your child's diet for more than three weeks, and the child won't drink soybean milk, you should check with your doctor about a calcium substitute. For more information on milk allergy see Adler 1976, Oski 1977, Prevention Magazine Editors 1972, Roth 1977, 1978, Sainsbury 1974, Conrad 1960, Emerling 1969, Frazier 1974, and Greer 1977.

CALCIUM REQUIREMENTS

Infant to 1 year—400 to 600 mg./day
Age 1 to 12 years—700 to 1200 mg./day
Age 12 to 18 years—1200 to 1400 mg./day
Cup milk = 288 mg. Ca/cup
Soybean milk = 200 mg. Ca/cup

CALCIUM SUBSTITUTES

Abbott Di-Cal-D—235 mg. each
2 to 12 years need 3 to 4 a day with meals
Sandoz-Neocalglucon (92 mg./tsp.)
Up to 7 years, 1 to 2 tsp. t.i.d.
Upjohn Calcium gluconate flavored wafers, 87 mg. each
Up to 1 year, 6 a day
Various nonchewable varieties are also available

If you want to find out if you have a milk allergy, try the following: First, eat only the *allowed* foods listed below for five to fourteen days. Notice if you are the same or better in any way when you are not drinking milk or eating milk-containing foods. Second, after you have stopped all milk products for two weeks (or sooner if you are perfectly well before then), start to eat dairy products and drink milk. When you re-add milk foods again, do your symptoms return? Check with your doctor if milk makes you worse in any way.

ALLOWED

Beverages
Carbonated beverages such as pop
Kool-Aid
Coffee Rich
Any soybean type milk (Isomil, Nursoy, Neo-Mull-Soy®)
Juice from canned fruits

FORBIDDEN

Beverages
Milk—cow's or goat's
Skim milk
2 percent milk
Buttermilk
Whole milk
Chocolate milk or drink
Malted milk
Coffee-mate
Dry milk
Evaporated milk
Powdered milk

Used by permission of Syntex Laboratories. From the booklet *Food Sensitivity Diets.*
© 1978 by Doris J. Rapp.

ALLOWED	FORBIDDEN

Milk Products

Allowed:
Margarines
  Diet Imperial
  Mother's
  Mrs. Filbert's Diet Spread
  Safflower
  Any Kosher "parve" brand
  Willow Run

Forbidden:
Butter
Casein or sodium caseinate
Cheese
Curds
Ice cream
Margarine (except those listed on left)
Whey
Cottage cheese
Yogurt

Fruits

Allowed: Any *fresh* fruit in any form

Forbidden: Read labels on all fruit desserts

Vegetables

Allowed: All allowed, except creamed

Forbidden: Any creamed type, i.e., corn, peas, etc.

Cereals

Allowed: All allowed if Coffee Rich, fruit juice, or soybean milk is used on top of cereal instead of milk

Forbidden:
Country Morning
Granola

Baked Goods

Allowed: Any providing they're not made with butter or any type of milk

Forbidden: Allow none if baked with butter or any type of milk. Allow no item with casein, sodium caseinate, or whey in ingredients

Breads

Allowed:
Rye breads (only the following):
  Grossman's
  Beefsteak
  Kaufman's
  Millbrook Swedish & Dixie Rye
  Arnold Jewish Rye
Italian breads (only the following):
  Balisteri's
  Kaufman's
  Maria's
  Marzolina's
  Ontario

Forbidden:
Eat only those listed on left
Do not eat
  Arnold
  Millbrook White
  Profile
  Tops
  Wonder
(Brand names vary in different parts of country—check with your doctor)

ALLOWED	FORBIDDEN

ALLOWED

Meats
All fresh meats
Kosher luncheon meats, hot dogs,
  bologna, and salami labeled
  "parve"
  Sinai brand
  Hebrew National (may be very
  spicy)
  "396"—all-beef hot dogs
All poultry without stuffing
All fish

Desserts and Snacks
Any providing they're not made
  with butter or any type of milk
Some examples:
  Abel's Bagels
  Ritz crackers
  Salerno saltines
  Stella D'oro Cookies
  Voovtman's Apple Oatmeal
  Cookies
Neo-Mull-Soy® Ice Cream
  (see recipe in section B4)

Miscellaneous
"Hershey's Special Bar"
Cocoa
  Hershey or Baker's bitter baking
  chocolate
Ontario bread crumbs
Any food labeled "parve" or
  "pareve"
Milk of Magnesia

FORBIDDEN

Meats
Non-Kosher luncheon meats
  Bologna
  Salami
  Wieners
  Sausage
  Meat loaf
  Cold cuts
Poultry with stuffing
Meat balls

Desserts and Snacks
Allow none that contain butter,
  milk, casein, sodium caseinate,
  or whey (which may be found in
  many)
Cookies
Candy (especially cremes,
  chocolate, opaque candy)
Chocolate (milk, some dark)
Ice cream and milk sherbet
Pudding
Waffle and biscuit mixes
Crackers (most snack crackers:
  saltines, Sara Lee, store brand,
  and Sunshine)

Miscellaneous
Au gratin foods
Creamed or scalloped foods
Gourmet foods w/cheese or milk
Gravy
Soups
White sauces

B6: **Diet to Check for Wheat Allergy**

If you want to find out if you have wheat allergy, try the following: First, eat only the *allowed* foods listed below for five to fourteen days. Notice if you are the same or better in any way when you are not eating wheat-containing foods. Second, check with your doctor after you have stopped wheat for two weeks (or sooner if you are completely well before then). When you re-add wheat, do your symptoms return? Check with your doctor if wheat makes you worse in any way.

For more information on wheat allergy see Adler 1976, Conrad 1960, Emerling and Jonckers 1969, Roth 1977, 1978, Prevention Magazine Editors 1972, Cottrell 1974, Greer 1977, and Wood 1972a, 1972b.

ALLOWED

Cereals
Any which do not contain wheat
    Corn (Corn Flakes)
    Rice (Rice Krispies, Puffed Rice)
    Oat
    Barley
    Soy
    Rye (grind up Ry-Krisp crackers
    or use Cream of Rye)

Beverages
Milk (regular, skim, 2 percent)
Fruit juice
Soybean milk
Buttermilk

Fruits and Vegetables
All fresh fruits and vegetables
Canned and frozen fruits and
    vegetables if not creamed, stewed
    or otherwise prepared with
    wheat

FORBIDDEN

Cereals
All which contain wheat (e.g.,
    Cream of Wheat, Farina, Grape-
    nuts, Puffed Wheat, Ralston's
    Shredded Wheat, Triscuits,
    Wheatena, Cheerios)

Beverages
Postum
Malted milk
Beer, ale
Wines (some)
Whiskies, gin
Coffee substitutes
Ovaltine

Fruits and Vegetables
Stewed fruits
Fruits contained in pies and jam
Creamed vegetables
Baked beans and chili con carne

ALLOWED

Baked Goods

Any which do not contain wheat
Use flours other than wheat, such
    as:
    Rice (muffins or bread)
    Barley
    Potato starch
    Oat
    Soya
Read Labels Carefully: All breads
    (rye, potato, etc.) usually contain
    wheat except Bavern Schnitten
    Rye Bread (Loblaw's)

Meats

All fresh meats, poultry, fish except
    those prepared with wheat (see
    right)

Desserts and Snacks

Any which do not contain wheat
    (see Baked Goods)
Jell-O
Fruit ice or sherbet

Soups

Any which do not contain wheat

FORBIDDEN

Baked Goods

Bread and breadcrumbs
Biscuits and biscuit mixes
Cakes, cake mixes, cake flour
Cookies
Crackers and cracker meal
Doughnuts and doughnut mixes
Melba toast
Pancake mixes
Pies and pastry
Popovers
Potato flour
Rusks
Rye bread
Waffles and waffle mixes
Yeast (except Fleischmann's)
Zwiebach

Meats

Breaded types
Canned
Swiss steak
Hot dogs and lunch meats
Premolded hamburger
Sausage
Meat loaf
Meat balls

Desserts and Snacks

(See Baked Goods)
Chocolate candy
Cheese spreads and sauces
Ice cream
Ice cream cones
Custards
Puddings
Sherbets

Soups

Most soups
    Campbell's tomato soup
    Bouillon cubes

ALLOWED	FORBIDDEN
	Soups (cont)
	Creamed soups
	Chowders
	Bisques

Miscellaneous	**Miscellaneous**
Instead of school lunches	Butter
Soups in Thermos (homemade)	Cream sauce
Fresh fruit	Dumplings
Vegetable wedges and sticks	Egg dishes (thickened with flour)
Ry-Krisp sandwiches	Fritters
Chicken drumsticks (not	Gravy
breaded)	Macaroni (noodles, ravioli,
Pork chops (not breaded)	spaghetti)
Potato chips (unadulterated)	Salad dressings
Fresh salad, fruit or vegetable	Scalloped dishes
Jell-O	Wheat germ
	No school lunches

To make all-purpose flour without wheat, mix

1 cup of cornstarch	3 cups of soya flour
2 cups of rice flour	3 cups of potato starch flour

Use equal amounts of this mixture to replace wheat flour in baking. Bake at a lower temperature for a longer period of time and the bread will be crustier.

To substitute for 1 cup of wheat flour, use

1⅛ cups of rolled oats or	⅝ cup of potato starch flour or
1 cup of rye meal or	⅞ cup of rice flour or
1¼ cups of rye flour or	½ cup of barley flour or
¾ cup of soya flour or	¾ cup of cornmeal

To substitute for 1 tablespoon of wheat flour as a thickening agent, you may use ½ tablespoon of cornstarch, potato starch flour, rice flour, or arrowroot flour, or you may use 2 teaspoons of quick tapioca.

B7: **Diet to Check for Sugar Allergy**

If you want to find out if you have a sugar allergy, try the following: First, eat only the *allowed* foods listed below for five to fourteen days. Keep an exact record of everything you eat during this period of time. Notice if you are the same, better, or worse in any way when you are not eating sugar or sugar products. Second, at the end of two weeks, or sooner, if you improve before fourteen days, eat as many sugar-containing items as possible. Notice in particular if you have any symptoms within an hour. If you do, see if Alka-Seltzer Antacid Formula without Aspirin helps. (Sugar sensitivities are often specific. You may find that only one or more of the following is a problem: corn, beet, cane, date, or maple sugar.) For more information on sugar allergy see Dworkin and Dworkin 1974, Cleave 1975, Duffy 1975, and Goldbeck and Goldbeck 1976.

ALLOWED	FORBIDDEN
Sweeteners	**Sweeteners**
Honey	Sugar—granulated, powdered,
Saccharin	brown, cane
Sucaryl—tablet and liquid	Corn syrup
Pure maple syrup	Store maple syrup
	Beet sugar
	Date sugar
Beverages	**Beverages**
Brewed coffee—without sugar	Instant coffee
Brewed tea—without sugar	Instant tea
Natural fruit juice:	Any presweetened drinks:
Mott's apple juice	Hi-C
Dole pineapple juice	Hawaiian Punch
Welch's grape juice	Kool-Aid (presweetened)
Tops orange juice	Carbonated soft drinks
Minute Maid orange juice	
Lincoln apple juice	
Cereals	**Cereals**
Cream of Wheat	Most cold cereals
Cream of Rice	Corn Flakes
Oatmeal	Rice Krispies
Puffed Wheat (plain)	Bran Flakes
Puffed Rice (plain)	Alpha Bits

Used by permission of Syntex Laboratories. From the booklet *Food Sensitivity Diets*.
© 1978 by Doris J. Rapp.

ALLOWED	FORBIDDEN
	Cereals (cont)
	All presweetened cereals
	"Natural" food cereals
Baked Goods	**Baked Goods**
All homemade	All commercial baked goods
Italian bread (most)	Snack crackers—most types
Italian rolls (most)	
Some soda crackers (Premium saltines)	
Ry-Krisp	
Fruits	**Fruits**
Fresh	Canned in corn syrup or sugar
Frozen (without syrup)	Sugared fresh fruit
	Frozen (in syrup)
Vegetables	**Vegetables**
Fresh	Most canned vegetables
Frozen	Candied sweet potatoes
Blue Boy canned vegetables	Creamed vegetables
	Instant potato flakes
Meats	**Meats**
Fresh cut meats	Hot dogs
Plain smoked meats	Ham (cured in syrup or sugar)
	Pork sausage
	Italian sausage
	Breakfast sausage
	Frozen prepared meats
	On-Cor beef
	Banquet fried chicken
	Bacon
Snacks	**Snacks**
Salted nuts	Candy
Raisins	Ice cream
Dried fruits without sugar	Sherbet
Sesame candy bars (health food store)	Cookies
Potato chips (no additives)	Snack crackers
Popsicles homemade from sugar-free fruit juice	

ALLOWED

Snacks (cont)
Toasted soy beans (health food
  store)
Ry-Krisp

Dairy Products
All milk, 2 percent skimmed,
  regular
Butter
Sour cream
Cottage cheese
Yogurt—plain
Milkshakes made with fruit and
  honey*
Brick cheese

*Recipe available from
AMERICAN HONEY INSTITUTE
  831 Union Street
  Shelbyville, TN 37160

Miscellaneous
Most tablet medicine
Mustard
Oil and vinegar dressing
Dietetic dressing
Horseradish
Homemade peanut butter
Toothpowder made from Sea salt
  and baking soda
Eggs

FORBIDDEN

Dairy Products
Processed cheese
Margarines
Ice cream
Sherbet
Fudgsicles
Chip dips
Flavored cottage cheese
Yogurt with fruit
Frozen milkshakes
Cheese sauces (commercial)

Miscellaneous
Most liquid medicine
Chewable tablets
Ketchup
Most bottled salad dressings
Canned soups
Commercial peanut butter
Toothpaste
Hershey cocoa syrup

PERCENTAGE OF SUGAR IN UNSUSPECTED FOOD ITEMS

Apple Jacks	56%	Sugar Pops	39%
Sugar Smacks	56%	Frosted Mini-Wheats	28%
Froot Loops	53%	Bran Buds	25%
Cocoa Krispies	46%	Country Morning	25%
Sugar Frosted Flakes	42%	Quaker 100% Natural	
Frosted Rice Krinkles	39%	cereal	23.9%

PERCENTAGE OF SUGAR (CONT)

Country Morning with		Sara Lee chocolate cake	35.9%
raisins, dates	21%	Wish-Bone Russian	
40% Bran	18%	dressing	30.2%
Pep	14%	Heinz ketchup	28.9%
Raisin Bran	14%	Sealtest chocolate ice	
All-Bran	14%	cream	21.4%
Concentrate	11%	Hamburger Helper	23%
Product 19	11%	Wish-Bone French	
Rice Krispies	11%	dressing	30.2%
Corn Flakes	7%	Cool Whip	21%
Special K	7%	Libby's peaches	17.9%
Jell-O	82.6%	Wyler's beef bouillon	
Coffee-mate	65.4%	cubes	14.8%
Cremora	56.9%	Dannon lowfat yogurt	13.7%
Hershey's chocolate bar	51.4%	Ritz crackers	11.8%
Shake 'n' Bake barbecue		Del Monte kernel corn	10.7%
chicken	50.9%	Skippy peanut butter	9.2%

B8: **Diet to Check for Egg Allergy**

If you want to find out if you have an egg allergy, try the following: First, eat only *allowed* foods listed below for five to fourteen days. Notice if you are the same or better in any way when you are not eating eggs or egg-containing foods. Second, after you have stopped eggs for two weeks (or sooner if you are perfectly well before then), begin to eat eggs and egg-containing foods again. When you re-add eggs, do your symptoms come back? Check with your doctor if eggs make you worse in any way.

ALLOWED

Egg Replacers
Jolly Joan Egg Replacer (See below)

Beverages
All except those listed on right

Fruits and Vegetables
Any type in any form (be careful of salad dressings containing eggs)

Baked Goods
Any which do not contain eggs in any form. "Jell-O" pie filling (vanilla and lemon may be egg-free)

FORBIDDEN

Eggs
Eggs in any form
Albumin
Egg white (meringue) and yolk
Powdered or dried egg
Fleischmann's Egg Beaters

Beverages
Coffee (if cleared with eggs—read label)
Egg nog
Root beer (some)
Ovaltine and Ovomalt

Fruits and Vegetables
All allowed
None with Hollandaise sauce

Baked Goods
Bavarian creams
Breads (especially with shiny crusts)
Cakes
Creamed pies
Doughnuts
Fritters
Meringue
Pancakes and waffles
Pie fillings (some)

Used by permission of Syntex Laboratories. From the booklet *Food Sensitivity Diets.* © 1978 by Doris J. Rapp.

ALLOWED	FORBIDDEN
Desserts and Snacks	**Desserts and Snacks**
Any which do not contain eggs in any form	Candy (most)
	Custards
	French ice cream
	Pretzels
	Pudding
Meats	**Meats**
All fresh meats, poultry, fish except those prepared with eggs and those listed on right	Fritter batter (fish)
	Sausages
	Egg dips used in breading liver, pork chops, chicken
Miscellaneous	**Miscellaneous**
Breakfast substitutes	Breadcrumbs (some)
Fruit	Creamed foods
Cereal (with juice from fruit, milk, or Coffee Rich)	Croquettes
Vegetables	French toast
Meat	Fritters
Homemade soup	Frosting
	Noodles
	Salad dressing
	Sauces (Hollandaise)
	Soups (noodle, consommes)
	Souffles
	Spaghetti

When baking, substitute ½ teaspoon of egg-free baking powder for each egg omitted from the recipe. Thus if the recipe calls for 2 teaspoons of baking powder and 2 eggs, you merely use 3 teaspoons of egg-free baking powder. Or you may use Jolly Joan Egg Replacer (health food store), substituting 1 teaspoon of the replacer plus 3 teaspoons of water for each egg. Thus if the recipe calls for two eggs, use 2 teaspoons of Jolly Joan Egg Replacer plus 6 teaspoons of water.

B9: **Diet to Check for Chocolate Allergy**

The general plan is to stop eating chocolate in any food or drink for a period of at least five to fourteen days. Is your child better in any way? The chocolate will then be re-added to the diet and your child will be encouraged to eat as much chocolate as possible to see if it seems to affect the nose, eyes, skin, chest, disposition, digestion, bed wetting, or activity. If chocolate in any form causes obvious symptoms, stop eating this food until you check with your doctor.

ALLOWED

Carob
CaraCoa*
Fruit juices or fruit beverages
Milk
Milk substitutes
  Soybean milk
  Coffee Rich

*For information about CaraCoa
substitute, write
EL MOLINO MILLS
  345 North Baldwin Park Blvd.
  City of Industry, CA 91746

FORBIDDEN

Any brown, green, pink, yellow or
  white chocolate
Any cola
  Pepsi-Cola
  Coca-Cola
  Diet-Cola
Chocolate in any
  Drink
  Candy
  Baked goods
    Cake
    Cookies
  Ice cream
Dorito's Taco Chips

Substitutes for chocolate which look and taste like chocolate but contain none are available at large grocery stores or health food stores. If some do not have an acceptable taste: 1 ounce chocolate = 3 tablespoons carob heated in 1 to 1½ tablespoons oil. Eat only the foods in the *allowed* list unless you already know your child is allergic to one of them.

Used by permission of Syntex Laboratories. From the booklet *Food Sensitivity Diets*.
© 1978 by Doris J. Rapp.

B10: Diet to Check for Dye or Food-Coloring Allergy

If you want to find out if you have a food-coloring sensitivity, try the following: First, eat and drink only the *allowed* foods listed below for five to fourteen days. Notice if you seem better in any way. If you have tried this diet for two weeks and are not better, it is doubtful that dyes are your problem. If you are much improved in less than a week see below. Second, if you seem improved in any way after eating only the *allowed* foods for one to two weeks, try eating a large number of the *forbidden* foods. Are you worse in any way? In particular notice your activity, disposition and behavior. Try Alka-Seltzer Antacid Formula without Aspirin if you seem worse, to see if it helps relieve your symptoms. Check with your physician at this point for his advice.

When you re-add food colors, be sure to take as many reds, blues, greens, yellows and oranges as possible. There are many food dye colors and only one may be a problem for some people. If you don't eat the right one, you may notice no effect. If you eat many colored items for three days and remain fine, dyes are probably not a problem for you. For more information about dye allergy see Lockey 1971, 1977, Hawley and Buckley, 1974a, b, and Green 1974.

ALLOWED

Cereals
Any natural type without any food coloring

Baked Goods
Any homemade types
Commercial baked goods if labeled dye-free

Meats
Most are all right except those at the right

FORBIDDEN

Cereals
Any colored type

Baked Goods
Most whole wheat breads
Any colored baked goods

Meats
Luncheon meats
Bologna
Salami
Kosher wieners
Some sausage
Some ham
Some hamburger

Used by permission of Syntex Laboratories. From the booklet *Food Sensitivity Diets.* © 1978 by Doris J. Rapp.

ALLOWED

Fish
All except those at the right

Vegetables
All, if fresh

Fruits
All fresh

Desserts
Homemade ice cream, pudding, or any item without any food coloring

Candy must be homemade

Beverages
Any labeled without food coloring
Grapefruit juice
Pineapple juice
Pear nectar
Guava nectar
Milk
Soybean milk
Coffee
Tea, if not colored
Homemade lemonade or limeade from fresh fruit
Some apple cider
Some orange juice
7up
Colorless creme soda

Miscellaneous
Some tub butter
Some cheese (white and specifically labeled)
Distilled white vinegar
Honey

FORBIDDEN

Fish
Frozen fish, dyed filets or sticks

Vegetables
Fresh frozen may be dyed and not so labeled
Avoid canned, unless specifically labeled "not dyed"

Fruits
Any frozen or canned unless specifically labeled "not dyed"

Desserts
Avoid gelatins, puddings, any box mixes, yogurt, sherbet, ice cream, or candy; unless label specifies "no food coloring"

Beverages
Kool-Aid
Colored pop or soda
Some frozen juices
All instant breakfast drinks
All powdered beverages
Coffee Rich (yellow dye)
Some tea mixes
Chocolate drinks or mixes

Miscellaneous
Most butter or margarine
Mustard
Soy sauce
Some vinegar
Ketchup

ALLOWED

Miscellaneous (cont)

Jam and jelly without food
 coloring—homemade
Homemade mayonnaise

Drugs and Other Items

If a colorless liquid or tablet or
 white pill without any color
 inside or outside
Drugs to treat allergy
 Liquid antihistamine (Tacaryl,
 Ryna)
 Liquid asthma drugs (Marax D F,
 Elixicon Suspension, Slo-Phyllin
 Syrup, Theospan Syrup)

FORBIDDEN

Miscellaneous (cont)

Chili or barbecue sauce
Some chocolate syrup
Most cheese

Drugs and Other Items

Most are colored in some way
Cough drops
Throat lozenges
Most toothpaste and mouthwash
Colored fluoride treatment
Colored dental cleaner

B11: **Diet to Check for Corn Allergy**

If you want to find out if you have a corn allergy, try the following: First, eat only the *allowed* foods listed below for five to fourteen days. Keep an exact record of everything you eat during this period of time. Notice if you are the same, better or worse in any way when you are not eating corn or corn products. Second, at the end of two weeks, or sooner if you improve before fourteen days, eat as many corn-containing foods as possible. Notice in particular if you have any symptoms within an hour. If you do, see if Alka-Seltzer Antacid Formula without Aspirin helps.

ALLOWED

Beverages or Drinks
Coffee—brewed (no instant)
Dole pineapple juice
Kool-Aid (sweetened with pure
  honey)
Milk—glass or plastic containers
Neo-Mull-Soy® formula,
  Nursoy, Isomil
Orange juice—Minute Maid
Tea—brewed
Tomato juice
Welch's grape juice (bottled)

Fruits
Any fresh fruits

Milk
All milk—if in glass
Cottage cheese
Butter

FORBIDDEN

Beverages or Drinks
Beer, ale, gin, whiskey
Canned or bottled juice drinks:
  Frozen orange juice—except
  Minute Maid
  Hawaiian Punch
  Hi-C
  Mott's apple juice
Coffee—instant
Coffee Rich
Infant formulas:
  Enfamil
  Evaporated milk
  SMA
  Similac
Some cranberry juice

Fruits
Candied fruits
Canned fruits
Dried fruits
Frozen fruits—sweetened
Fruit desserts

Milk
Cheese—none except cottage cheese
Ice cream
No milk in paper containers

Used by permission of Syntex Laboratories. From the booklet *Food Sensitivity Diets.*
© 1978 by Doris J. Rapp.

ALLOWED	FORBIDDEN
	Milk (cont)
	Oleomargarine
	Sherbet
	Yogurt

Vegetables

ALLOWED: Any fresh ones

FORBIDDEN:
Corn
Hominy — neither canned, creamed, or frozen
Succotash

Baked Goods

FORBIDDEN:
All commercial baked goods
Biscuits
Bisquick
Cake mixes
Cookies
Doughnuts
Golden Mix
Pancake mixes
Pie crusts
Py-O-My

ALLOWED: Homemade

Cereals

ALLOWED — Non-presweetened types such as:
    Cream of Wheat
    Oatmeal
    Puffed Rice
    Rice Chex
    Rice Krispies
    Wheat Chex
    Wheaties

FORBIDDEN:
Alpha Bits
Cheerios
Corn Flakes
Grits
Pablum
Post Toasties
All presweetened cereals
Sugar-coated rice cereals

Bread

ALLOWED: Homemade with special ingredients (Corn-free baking powders and yeast)

FORBIDDEN: All commercial breads

Meats

ALLOWED	FORBIDDEN
Beef	Bacon
Chicken	Cooked meats in gravies
Pork	Ham—cured
Veal	Luncheon meats (bologna, etc.)

ALLOWED

FORBIDDEN

Meats (cont)
Sandwich spreads
Sausages
Wieners

Sweeteners
Beet sugar*
Honey**
Pure maple sugar
Saccharin

Sweeteners
Brown sugar
Cane sugar
Confectioner's sugar
Corn sugars
Corn syrup
Sorbitol

*Not available in upper New York
State
**Bake or make candy with
honey instead of sugar. (1 cup
honey = 1 cup sugar, but liquid
must be reduced by ¼ cup. For
example, for a recipe for 1 cup of
sugar and 1 cup of milk, use 1 cup
honey and ¾ cup milk.) For further information:
AMERICAN HONEY INSTITUTE
831 Union Street
Shelbyville, TN 37160

Desserts and Snacks
Baker's chocolate
Candy made with honey
Cocoa
Freshly ground peanut butter
Hershey's chocolate
Maple candy—pure
Ry-Krisp

Desserts and Snacks
Candy
Carob (CaraCoa)
Creamed pies
Cookies
Custards
Frostings
Fritos
Graham crackers
Ice cream
Jellies
Jell-O
Peanut butter
Popcorn
Puddings
Sherbet

ALLOWED	FORBIDDEN

Baking Ingredients

Baking Ingredients	**Baking Ingredients**
Baking powder—(corn free)	All usual baking powders
Ditex baking powder	All corn oils (Mazola)
Red Star dry yeast	All yeast (except Red Star dry yeast)
Wesson oil	Corn meal
Safflower oil	Corn starch
Tapioca	
Unbleached flour	
Safflower oil	

Medicines	**Medicines**
Actifed	Aspirin
Antihistamines	Bufferin
Cecom	Capsules
Cyrobeta	Ointments
Histadyl	Suppositories
Upjohn's allergic line of drugs	Most tablet or pill medicine
Vitamin B	Some vitamins
Vitamin C	

Miscellaneous

ALLOWED

Use Wesson Oil (cottonseed) or any type which is not corn

Use tapioca or flour instead of corn starch for a thickening agent for gravies

Try to avoid all obvious and hidden sources of corn

Read all labels

FORBIDDEN

Miscellaneous

Inhalants
  No bath or body powders
  Cooking, fumes of popcorn or fresh corn
Paper cups and plates
Adhesives
  Envelopes
  Labels
  Stickers
  Tapes
  Stamps
Liquids from paper cartons
Some plastic food wrappers
Toothpaste/powder
Foods fried in corn oil
Gravies
Monosodium glutamate
Zest soap
Sorbitol

B12: **Citrus-Free Diet**

Some patients are allergic to citrus and others to citric acid. These lists may help you determine if you are allergic to either or both.

ALLOWED

Non-Citrus Fruits and Juices
Apple (bottled)
Grape (Welch's juice)
Prune (bottled)
Cranberry (bottled)
Pear (bottled)
Peach (bottled)
Apricot (bottled)
Pineapple (bottled)
Tomato (bottled)

Beverages
Cola
Cherry pop
Root beer
Vegetable juice

Miscellaneous
Popsicles
  Grape
  Root beer
  Banana

FORBIDDEN

Citrus Fruits and Juices
Orange
Grapefruit
Lemon
Lime
Kumquat
Tangerine

Beverages
Soda pop (7up, Squirt, Teem,
  Uptown)
Kool-Aid
Hi-C
Constant Comment Tea

Miscellaneous
Medicines
  Liquids
  Tablets
  Flavor-coated pills
  Lozenges
  Cough drops
Desserts
  Jell-O
  Candy and gum
  Sherbet

Check all labels carefully for foods containing citrus—if in doubt, don't eat. If a food contains "citric acid" it may not necessarily contain citrus. However, some patients are allergic to both citric acid and citrus and must avoid both.

Used by permission of Syntex Laboratories. From the booklet *Food Sensitivity Diets*.
© 1978 by Doris J. Rapp.

B13: **Citric-Acid-Free Diet**

ALLOWED

Fruits and Juices
Apple (bottled, not canned)
Banana
Cherry (bottled, not canned)
Grape (Welch's juice, not drink, not
  frozen)
Cranberry
Prune
Pear
Peach
Apricot

Beverages and Desserts
Cola
Cherry pop
Root beer (Shasta)
Vegetable juice

Miscellaneous
Popsicles
  Root beer
  Banana
Some medicines
Some candy
Some cough drops

FORBIDDEN

Fruits and Juices
Oranges
Grapefruit
Lemon
Lime
Pineapple
Tomato
Kumquats
Tangerines

Beverages and Desserts
Jell-O
Suckers
Pop (7up, Squirt, Teem, Uptown)
Sherbet
Candy, gum
Baked goods
Kool-Aid
Hi-C

Miscellaneous
Medicines
  Liquids
  Vitamins
  Tablets
  Flavor-coated pills
  Lozenges
  Cough drops
Snacks (e.g., Munchos)
Alka-Seltzer Antacid Formula
  without Aspirin

Check all labels for citric-acid-containing foods. If in doubt, do not eat. A beverage labeled "drink" such as "grape drink" means citric acid has been added. Foods containing acids other than citric, for instance, ascorbic acid (vitamin C) are OK.

Used by permission of Syntex Laboratories. From the booklet *Food Sensitivity Diets*. © 1978 by Doris J. Rapp.

B14: **Common Sources of Pork Contact**

FRESH PORK

Pork roast
Pork chops
Pork sausage (dried or smoked venison, German, etc.)
Pork liver

Pork brains
Pork kidneys
Crackling or chitterlings (chitlings)
Souse (head cheese)
Ribs, spare—barbecue

CURED PORK

Bacon, vegetables with bacon drippings, soups, pork and beans
Ham, vegetable stock, salads
Sausage

Pickled pig's feet (souse)
Rinds (like potato chips)
Salt pork

PROCESSED PORK

Wieners
Vienna Sausage
Luncheon meats
Liverwurst

Mincemeat
Spam
Canned meats such as "potted" meats

DERIVATIVES OF PORK

Lard, bacon drippings, shortening, margarine, vegetable stock
Mayonnaise, salad dressing
Instant foods: mashed potatoes, puddings, prepared cake and pancake mixes, frosting mixes
Prebreaded frozen foods: frozen seafood and fish
Fried foods: French fries and fried foods in restaurants
Vegetables seasoned with salt pork
Nondairy cream, Coffee-mate, etc; glue in milk carton
Mexican food (tortillas, etc.) and Chinese and Polynesian foods
Potato chips, Fritos, etc.
Candy bars
Ice cream
Gelatin, Jell-O, etc.

Bakery products: breads, cakes, cookies, pastries, soda crackers, doughnuts (read labels carefully)
Drugs: thyroid tablets, ACTH, capsules, tonics and pills for anemia (hog stomach is intrinsic factor), calcium and magnesium stearates
Glycerin: Soaps, cosmetics, sometimes in processed cheeses in jars and cartons, cocktail dips, etc.
Glue
Other: Iron skillets and Dutch ovens which have not been thoroughly scoured after using to cook pork.
Soaps

This list is used with the kind permission of Dor Brown, M.D., of Fredericksburg, Texas.

B15: **Common Sources of Yeast Contact**

The following foods contain yeast as an additive ingredient in preparation (often called leavening):

Breads
Crackers
Pastries
Pretzels
Hamburger buns
Hot dog buns
Cake and cake mix
Rolls, homemade or canned
Canned ice box biscuits:
  Borden, Pillsbury, and General
  Mills

Cookies
Flour enriched with vitamins from
  yeast
  General Mills, Inc.
  Flour Corporation flour and
    enrichment wafers
  Pfizer Laboratories enrichment
    products
  Hungarian Flour Mills
Milk fortified with vitamins
Meat fried in cracker crumbs
Salt-rising bread

The following substances contain yeast or yeastlike substances, because of their nature or the nature of their manufacture or preparation.

Morel mushrooms, truffles, and cheese of all kinds including cottage cheese, buttermilk, sour cream, soy sauce, black tea, sour dough
All vinegars: apple, pear, grape, and distilled. These may be used as such or they will be used in these foods: ketchup, mayonnaise, olives, pickles, sauerkraut, condiments, horse-radish, French dressing, salad dressing, barbecue sauce, tomato sauce, chili peppers
All fermented beverages: whiskey, wine, brandy, gin, rum, vodka, root beer, ginger ale, beer

All malted products: cereals, candy, and milk drinks which have been malted
All citrus fruit juices, whether frozen or canned. Only home-squeezed are yeast free
All dried fruits (e.g., prunes, raisins, dates, etc.)
Antibiotics: Penicillin, Mycin drugs, Chloromycetin, B_{12}, Tetracyclines, Lincocin and any other derived from mold culture. (Meat from animals given antibiotics.)
Some monosodium glutamate may be a yeast derivative
Citric acid—almost always a yeast derivative

This list is used with the kind permission of Dor Brown, M.D., of Fredericksburg, Texas.

164

The following substances are derived from yeast or have their source from yeast:

Vitamin B capsules or tablets, if made with yeast

Multiple vitamins, capsules or tablets with vitamin B made from yeast

Zylax, Zymelose, Zymenol, vitamin products which contain B_{12}

U.S. vitamin products:
Laxo-Funk
Phoscaron-D
Vi-Litron Drops
Mead Johnson's vitamins which contain B_{12}

Squibb's vitamin products if indicated on the label.

Parke Davis's vitamin product: Vibex

Merck, Sharp & Dohme vitamin products which contain B_{12}

Lederle's vitamin products

Endo's vitamin products

Manibee tablets, S.C.T.

Massengill vitamins

Citric acid

The following products are known to be free of yeast as of November 1970

Ritz crackers
Pioneer Flour Mills
Gladiola Flour Mills
International Flour Mills
Archway Baker products (if ingredients otherwise allowed)
Vemp Flour
El Molino flour

Royal Crest-Pasteurized Cream Top
Regular Quaker Oats
Plain rice
Corn meal
Cream of Rye
Shurfine Puffed Rice
Wheatena
Buckwheat

Almost all vitamins contain yeast as well as the following:

Gelseal Eprolin
Ampoule Betalin
  B_{12} Crystalline

Tablets: Folic Acid
Tablets: Pantholin
Tablets: Riboflavin
Tablets: Rutin

Read labels very thoroughly. It is possible additions can be found to this list.

B16: **The K-P Diet (Feingold)**

This diet consists of the elimination of two groups of foods at the same time.

Group 1

This is a group of fruits and vegetables which contain natural salicylates. They must be omitted in all forms: fresh, frozen, canned, dried or juice or as an ingredient of prepared foods.

Fruits

Almonds
Apples
Apricots
Berries
    Blackberries
    Boysenberries
    Gooseberries
    Raspberries
    Strawberries
Cherries
Currants
Grapes and raisins or any products
    made of grapes: wine, wine
    vinegar, jellies, etc.
Nectarines
Oranges (Note: grapefruits, lemons,
    and limes are allowed)
Peaches
Plums and prunes

Vegetables

Tomatoes and all tomato products
Cucumbers (pickles)
Green peppers

From Ben F. Feingold, *Why Your Child Is Hyperactive* (Random House) pp., 169 to 175. © 1975 by Ben F. Feingold, used by permission.

Group 2

The foods omitted in Group 2 contain artificial color and flavor. BHT or butylated hydroxytoluene must also be omitted. Be sure to read every detail of every label.

ALLOWED

Cereals

Any cereal without artificial colors or flavors, dry or cooked

Bakery Goods

Any product without artificial color or flavor, but most bakery items must be prepared at home
All commercial breads except eggbread and whole wheat (usually dyed)
All flours

All Meats

Except those to the right

Poultry

All poultry except stuffed and those to the right

Fish

All fresh fish except those to the right

FORBIDDEN

Cereals

All cereals with artificial colors and flavors
All instant-breakfast preparations

Bakery Goods

All manufactured cakes, cookies, pastries, sweet rolls, doughnuts, etc.
Pie crusts
Frozen baked goods
Many packaged baking mixes

Luncheon Meats

Bologna
Salami
Frankfurters
Sausages*
Meat loaf or balls
Ham, bacon, pork*

*When colored or flavored, usually indicated on the package.

Poultry

All barbecued types
All turkeys with prepared basting, called "self-basting," prepared stuffing

Fish

Frozen fish filets that are dyed or flavored; fish sticks that are dyed or flavored

ALLOWED

Desserts

Homemade ice cream without
artificial coloring or flavoring
Gelatins—homemade from pure
gelatins with any permitted
natural fruit or fruit juices
Tapioca
Homemade custards and puddings
Plain yogurt

Candies

Homemade candies, without
almonds or nut flavoring

Beverages

Grapefruit juice
Pineapple juice
Pear nectar
Guava nectar
Homemade lemonade or limeade
from fresh lemons or limes
7up
Milk

Miscellaneous

All cooking oils and fats
Sweet butter, not colored or
flavored
Mustard prepared at home from
pure powder and distilled
vinegar
Jams or jellies made from permitted
fruits, not artificially colored or
flavored
Honey
Homemade mayonnaise
Distilled white vinegar
Homemade chocolate syrup for all
purposes
All natural (white) cheeses

FORBIDDEN

Desserts

Manufactured ice creams, unless
the label specifies no synthetic
coloring or flavoring; the same
applies to sherbet, ices, gelatins,
junkets, puddings
All powdered puddings
All dessert mixes
Flavored yogurt

Candies

All manufactured types, hard or
soft

Beverages

Cider
Wine
Beer
Diet drinks
Soft drinks
All instant-breakfast drinks
All quick-mix powdered drinks
Tea, hot or cold
Prepared chocolate milk

Miscellaneous

Oleomargarine
Colored butter
Mustard
All mint-flavored items
Soy sauce, if flavored or colored
Cider vinegar
Wine vinegar
Commercial chocolate syrup
Barbecue-flavored potato chips
Cloves
Ketchup
Chili sauce
Colored cheese

Dr. Ben F. Feingold stresses that BHT and BHA may be as important as
dyes in relation to hyperkinesis (see appendix B17).

B17: **Common Food Additives**

CLASS OR TYPE OF FOOD ADDITIVES

Nutrient Supplements
Thiamine (vitamin B_1)
Riboflavin (vitamin B_2)
Niacin (vitamin B_3)
Iron
Vitamin A
Vitamin D
Potassium iodide

Nonnutritive Sweeteners
Saccharin
Calcium and sodium cyclamates
  (cyclo hexyl sulfamates)

Preservatives
Antioxidants (for fatty products)
  BHA (butylated hydroxyanisole,
    see below)
  BHT (butylated hydroxytolu-
    ene, see below)
  NDGA (nordihydroguaiaretic
    acid)
  Propyl gallate
  Mold or Rope Inhibitors or
    Antimycotic Agents
  Sodium and calcium propionate
  Sodium diacetate
  Lactic acid
  Sorbic acids
  Sodium and potassium sorbates
  Fungicides
Sequestrants
  Sodium, calcium and potassium
  salts of citric
  Tartaric, metaphosphoric, and
  pyrophosphoric acids

Other
Benzoic acid
Sodium benzoate, sulfur dioxide

Emulsifiers
Lecithin
Mono and diglycerides
Propylene glycol alginate

Stabilizers and Thickeners
Pectins
Vegetable gums (carob bean,
  carrageenan, guar)
Gelatin
Agar agar

Acids, Alkalies, Buffers, Neutralizing Agents
Ammonium bicarbonate
Calcium carbonate
Potassium acid tartrate
Sodium aluminum phosphate
Tartaric acid

Flavoring Agents
Amyl acetate
Benzaldehyde
Ethyl butyrate
Methyl salicylate
Essential oils
Monosodium glutamate

Bleaching Agents: Bread Improvers
Benzoyl peroxide
Oxides of nitrogen
Chlorine dioxide
Nitrosyl chloride
Chlorine
Potassium bromate
Ammonium chloride
Calcium sulfate
Ammonium phosphates
Calcium phosphates

This list is used with the kind permission of James O'Shea, M.D.

169

BHT—BUTYLATED HYDROXYTOLUENE FOOD ADDITIVE

Type	Specified Uses
Antioxidant	In potato flakes
	In chewing gum base
	In dry breakfast cereals
	In emulsion stabilizers for shortenings
	In sweet potato flakes
	In potato granules
	In lard and shortening
Antifoaming agent	Used in processing beet sugar and yeast
Preservative	Enriched rice

This list is used with the kind permission of Stephen Lockey, MD. © 1978.

BHA—BUTYLATED HYDROXYANISOLE FOOD ADDITIVE

Type	Specified Use
Preservative—Antioxidant	In dry mixes for beverages and desserts
	In beverages and desserts prepared from dry mixes
	In active dry yeast
Antioxidant	In lard and shortening
	In unsmoked dry sausage
	In chewing gum base
	In dry breakfast cereals
	In emulsion stabilizers for shortenings
	In sweet potato flakes
	In mixed, diced, glazed fruits
	In potato granules
	In potato flakes
Antifoaming Agent	Defoaming agent component (used in processing beet sugar and yeast as an antioxidant)

This list is used with the kind permission of Stephen Lockey, M.D. © 1978.

B18: **Dr. Crook's Rare Food Diet**

Avoid any and every food on this list which you normally eat more often than once a week. Do this diet for five to ten days. Always stay on the diet two days after you're sure it's helping. Then add back foods, one at a time to identify troublemakers. Avoid all foods not on this list.

Vegetables

Asparagus	Onions	Cucumber
Cauliflower	Turnips	Okra
Brussels sprouts	Collards	Carrots
Radishes	Rutabaga	Squash
Beets	Broccoli	Sweet potatoes
Celery	Cabbage	Kale
Eggplant	Sauerkraut	Avocado
Green pepper	Mushrooms	Greens (beet, mustard, spinach, turnip)

Fruits

Most canned fruits are packed in "heavy" or "light" syrup. Such syrup contains cane and corn sugar, so you can't use them on this diet. Instead, get water-packed fruits or juices, or those packed in their own juice.

Pears	Peaches	Nectarines
Cranberries	Apricots	Raspberries
Cantaloupe	Strawberries	Dewberries
Dates	Blackberries	Boysenberries
Cherries	Loganberries	Grapes
Blueberries	Bananas	Pineapple
Watermelon	Figs	Raisins
Coconut	Persimmons	Blueberries
Plums	Prunes	

Meats

Avoid *processed meats*, such as salami, wieners, etc., since they often contain milk solids, corn syrup, dextrose, cane sugar, and food coloring. Commercially available *frozen turkeys* are basted with corn oil or milk and must be avoided. Some *canned fish* are canned in vegetable oil, which may be corn oil and should be avoided. Get fish packed in water or its own oil.

Used with permission of William G. Crook, M.D. From *Tracking Down Hidden Food Allergy* (Jackson, Tenn.: Professional), © 1978 by William G. Crook.

Lamb	Turkey
Duck	Frozen raw fish
Fresh fish	Canned salmon
Canned tuna	Clams
Oysters	Lobster
Shrimp	Squirrel
Sardines	Crab
Rabbit	Game birds
Goose Quail	

Breads, Cakes, Crackers. Because wheat, corn, and other grains are such common causes of chronic allergy, it is best for you to avoid all grains while on this diet. Sometimes your doctor may allow you to have breads and crackers made from oat or rice flours. If this is the case, you will usually need to bake your own, since commercial products contain wheat. You can also use arrowroot flour.

Beverages. Water, pineapple juice, tomato juice, herb tea.

Miscellaneous. Nuts: Cashews, pistachios, almonds, Brazil nuts, English walnuts, black walnuts, hickory nuts, pecans, butternuts, chestnuts, and hazel nuts; no peanuts. Do not eat any nuts from a can of mixed nuts. Use nuts in the shell or from the health food store, since many commercially available nuts contain vegetable oils, dextrose, and other additives.

Detailed instructions for carrying out the Rare Food Diet can be found in *Tracking Down Hidden Food Allergy* (1978, $4.50) available from
PROFESSIONAL BOOKS
Box 3494
Jackson, TN 38301

Appendix C · Resources

C1: **Organizations to Help Patients with Nervous System Allergies Due to Food, Water, or Air**

HUMAN ECOLOGY ACTION LEAGUE—HEAL
4054 McKinney Avenue
Suite 310
Dallas, TX 75204
This national organization has two publications, one for education; the other for legislative action. They disseminate information about ecology and support research in this area.

THE HUMAN ECOLOGY RESEARCH FOUNDATION
720 N. Michigan Avenue
Chicago, IL 60611
This foundation supports ecologic research and supplies reprints of articles pertaining to nervous-system problems, obesity, alcoholism, mental illness, and the effects of insecticides.

FEINGOLD ASSOCIATION OF THE UNITED STATES, INC.
Vickie L. Gelardi, President
1029 Jericho Turnpike
Smithtown, NY 11787
(516) 543-4658

ALLERGY INFORMATION ASSOCIATION
Room 7
25 Poynter Drive
Weston, Ontario, Canada M9R 1K8
This group has regular meetings to share information, plus a newsletter and diet lists.

NEW ENGLAND FOUNDATION FOR ALLERGIC AND ENVIRONMENTAL DISEASE
3 Brush Street
Norwalk, CT 06850
Nonprofit organization with publications available concerning effects of air pollution, mental illness, obesity, food problems, and hypoglycemia.

ALLERGY FOUNDATION OF LANCASTER COUNTY
Box 1424
Lancaster, PA 17604

Most informative nonprofit organization with publications available with elimination lists for patients sensitive to aspirin, antihistamines, barbiturates, natural penicillin, iodine, phenophthalein, sulfonamides, tetracyclines, mercury, food and alcohol, additives, salicylates, and dyes.

GROWTH INSTITUTES, INC.
124 North Clara
Deland, FL 32720

This is a center for nutrition, learning, and behavior. The emphasis is on the diagnosis and rapid training of parents to work with children in their own home when the children have learning and behavior problems. They are primarily interested in the family in relation to the child.

C2: Organizations to Help Patients with Learning Disabilities

ASSOCIATION FOR CHILDREN WITH LEARNING DISABILITIES—ACLD
4156 Library Road
Pittsburgh, PA 15234
This organization has branches throughout the United States to help parents and children in the school and community. They publish a monthly newspaper.

THE ORTON SOCIETY, INC.
Box 153
Pomfret, CT 06258
A nonprofit organization to study, prevent, and treat specific language disabilities, such as dyslexia. It publishes annually.

CALIFORNIA ASSOCIATION FOR NEUROLOGICALLY HANDICAPPED CHILDREN—CANHC
P.O. Box 604
Main Office
Los Angeles, CA 90053
They welcome members from any state and publish a regular newsletter.

THE READING REFORM FOUNDATION
6054 East Indian School Road
Scottsdale, AZ 85251
They publish aids to help parents teach children to read phonetically.

CANADIAN ASSOCIATION FOR CHILDREN WITH LEARNING DISABILITIES—CACLD
88 Eglington Avenue
Suite 322
Toronto, 315, Canada

THE QUEBEC ASSOCIATION FOR CHILDREN WITH LEARNING DISABILITIES
4820 Van Horne Avenue
Room 8
Montreal, Quebec H3W 1J3, Canada
A very active group with many instructive, informative, and referral services.

SOCIETY FOR EMOTIONALLY DISTURBED CHILDREN—SEDC
1622 Sherbrooke West
Montreal, H3H 1O9, Canada
This is another group to help parents and children by conferences, and publications (books, pamphlets, and paperbacks).

175

C3: **Physicians Practicing Ecology**

Physicians practicing ecology are both interested in and trained in, to varying degrees, the diagnosis and therapy of health problems which appear related to foods and various types of environmental contamination or pollution. They believe that susceptible individuals of all ages can have adverse reactions to natural and unnatural exposures in our food, water, air, drugs, and homes. These doctors believe such exposures can cause maladaptation in afflicted persons, which can manifest in a wide variety of intermittent or constant, acute or chronic, physical or mental symptoms. They stress avoidance and dietary manipulation, rather than drug therapy. Many treat patients using various forms of allergy-extract therapy if the patient does not respond to the above.

The society was founded in 1965 by a number of pioneers in this field which included French Hansel, Herbert Rinkel, Jonathan Forman, Carlton Lee, Theron Randolph, George Frauenberger, and Francis Silver. The growing membership includes a wide variety of medical and other specialists who recognize and appreciate the scope of this type of problem in our society. Names of physicians who are ecologists in your area will be provided.

SOCIETY FOR CLINICAL ECOLOGY
Del Stigler
1750 Humboldt St.
Denver, CO 80218

Names of ear and eye specialists familiar with food testing and therapy will be provided through:

THE AMERICAN SOCIETY OF OPHTHALMOLOGIC AND OTOLARYNGOLOGIC ALLERGY
William P. King, M.D., Secretary
1415 Third Street
Corpus Christi, TX 78404

C4: **Book Sources**

Academic Therapy Publications, 1539 Fourth Street, San Rafael, CA 94901
Allergy, Toxins & the Learning Disabled Child, $4.00
The Orthomolecular Approach to Learning Disabilities
Acropolis Books, Colortone Building, 2400 17th Street, N.W., Washington, DC 20009
How to Live With Your Special Child, $7.50
Arco Publishing Co., Inc., 219 Park Avenue South, New York, NY 10003
The Pulse Test, $1.95
Bantam Books, Dept. NN, 414 E. Golf Rd., Des Plaines, IL 60016
Consumer Beware (Your Food and What's Been Done to It), $1.95
Barnes & Noble Books, 10 E. 53 St., New York, NY 10022
The Allergy Cookbook, $2.50
Charles C Thomas, 301 East Lawrence Avenue, Springfield, IL 62703
Delicious and Easy Rice Flour Recipes, $3.75
Basics of Food Allergy, $29.00
Food Allergy and the Allergic Patient: A Simple Review of Problems Encountered by the Recently Diagnosed Patient, $4.50
Gourmet Food on a Wheat-Free Diet or Delicious and Easy Rice Recipes, $6.00
Understanding Allergies, $3.95
Allergy and Immunology in Children, $39.50
Food Allergy: Provocative Testing and Injection Therapy, $11.75
Allergy of the Nervous System, $14.00
Human Ecology and Susceptibility to the Chemical Environment, $9.25
Clinical Ecology, $35.75
The Milk-Free and Milk-Free, Egg-Free Cookbook, $8.95
Case Studies in Hyperactivity (in press)
Contemporary, 180 N. Michigan Ave., Chicago, IL 60601
Cooking for Your Hyperactive Child, $10.95
The Food Depression Connection, $9.95
Devin-Adair Co., Inc., 143 Sound Beach Avenue, Old Greenwich, CT 06870
Please, Doctor, Do Something, $6.95
Trace Elements & Man, $8.00
Drake Publishing, 381 Park Avenue South, New York, NY 10016
Questions and Answers About Allergies and Your Child, $4.95
Errand Press Ltd., Southsea, Hants, England
Copies from: Rita Greer, 44 Wallisdean Avenue, Portsmouth, England
The First Clinical Ecology Cookbook, $6.50

G.P. Putnam's Sons, 200 Madison Avenue, New York, NY 10016
  The Doctor's Book of Vitamin Therapy, $7.95
Grosset & Dunlap, 51 Madison Avenue, New York, NY 10010
  Psycho-nutrition, $7.95
  Live Longer Now . . . The First 100 Years of Your Life, $7.95
  The Healing Factor, $2.00
Harcourt Brace Jovanovich, 757 Third Avenue, New York, NY 10017
  Something is Wrong With My Child, $8.95
  Eating Dangerously, $6.95
Harper & Row Publishers, Inc., 10 E. 53rd Street, New York, NY 10022
  Raising the Hyperactive Child, $10.95
  The Psychobiology of Aggression, $12.95
Holt Rinehart & Winston, 383 Madison Avenue, New York, NY 10017
  Allergies and Your Child, $7.00
Human Ecology Foundation of Canada, 206 St. James St. So, Hamilton, Ontario L8P 3A9
  Common Sense for the Sensitive, $8.00
Human Ecology Research Foundation, 720 N. Michigan Avenue, Chicago, IL 60611
  Air Pollution in the Schools and Its Effect on Our Children, $1.50
Human Ecology Study Group, Fort Collins, CO 80521
  Very Basically Yours Cookbook, $5.00
Indiana University Press, Tenth and Morton Streets, Bloomington, IN 47401
  The Poisons Around Us (Toxic Metals in Food, Air and Water), $6.95
Johnny Reads, Inc., Box 12834, St. Petersburg, FL 33733
  Allergy, Brains and Children Coping, $7.00
Little, Brown & Co., 34 Beacon Street, Boston, MA 02106
  Square Pegs—Round Holes, $7.50
Keats Publishing Co., 36 Grove Street, New Canaan CT 06840
  The Saccharin Disease, $5.50
  The Fact Book on Food Additives and Your Health, $1.25
  Mental and Elemental Nutrients, $10.00
Naturegraph Publications, Happy Camp, CA 96039
  Beyond the Staff of Life, paperback $3.00, clothbound $7.00
New American Library, 1301 Avenue of the Americas, New York, NY 10019
  The Supermarket Handbook, $2.25
New England Foundation of Allergic and Environmental Diseases, 3 Brush Street, Norwalk, CT 06850
  Food Allergy, $11.00
  Management of Complex Allergies, $10.00
Pergamon Press, Inc., Fairview Park, Elmsford, NY 10523

A Physician's Handbook on Orthomolecular Medicine, $16.50
Peter H. Wyden Publishers, 750 Third Avenue, New York, NY 10017
  Meganutrients for Your Nerves, $11.95
  Don't Drink Your Milk, $9.95
Pocket Books, 1230 Avenue of the Americas, New York, NY 10020
  Health & Light, $1.95
Professional Books, P.O. Box 3494, Jackson, TN 38301
  Can Your Child Read? Is He Hyperactive?, $4.95
  Are You Allergic?, $3.95
  Tracking Down Hidden Food Allergy, $2.50
Pyramid Books, 919 Third Avenue, New York, NY 10022
  Allergy Cooking, $.95
Quadrangle/The New York Times Book Co., 10 E. 53 Street, New York,
  NY 10022
  Coping with Food Allergy, $9.95
Random House, 201 E. 50th Street, New York, NY 10022
  Why Your Child Is Hyperactive, $7.95
Rodale Press, Emmaus, PA 18049
  Natural Cooking the Prevention Way, $4.95
  Natural Snacks 'n' Sweets, $4.95
Simon & Schuster Publishing Co., 1230 Avenue of the Americas, New
  York, NY 10020
  Coping With Your Allergies, $9.95
Stein & Day, 7 East 48th Street, New York, NY 10017
  Psychodietetics, $7.95
Upjohn Co., Kalamazoo, Michigan
  Physical Signs of Allergy of the Respiratory Tract in Children, $4.00
Van Nostrand Reinhold Co., 450 W. 33rd Street, New York, NY 10001
  *The Ecologic-Biochemical Approaches to Treatment of Delinquents and
  Criminals,* $16.95
Vintage Press, see Random House
  Food for Nought, $3.95
Wacker, John A., Box 20445, Dallas, TX 75220
  *The Reduction of Crime Thru the Prevention and Treatment of Learning
  Disabilities,* no charge
Warner Books, 75 Rockefeller Plaza, New York, NY 10019
  Sugar Blues, $1.95
Williams and Wilkins Co., Inc., 428 E. Preston Street, Baltimore, MD
  21202
  *Deviant Children Grow Up: A Sociological and Psychiatric Study of
  Sociopathic Personality,* $13.50
Woodridge Press, Santa Barbara, CA 93111
  Oats, Peas, Beans, Barley, $4.50

Appendix D · Pollen Calendar

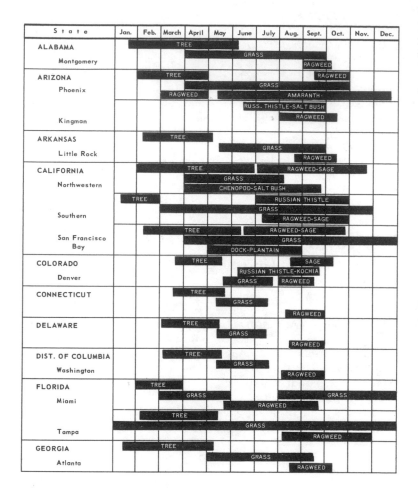

State	Jan.	Feb.	March	April	May	June	July	Aug.	Sept.	Oct.	Nov.	Dec.
ALABAMA			TREE									
Montgomery						GRASS			RAGWEED			
ARIZONA			TREE						RAGWEED			
Phoenix						GRASS			AMARANTH			
			RAGWEED				RUSS. THISTLE-SALT BUSH					
Kingman							RUSS. THISTLE-SALT BUSH		RAGWEED			
ARKANSAS			TREE									
Little Rock						GRASS			RAGWEED			
CALIFORNIA				TREE			RAGWEED-SAGE					
Northwestern					GRASS							
					CHENOPOD-SALT BUSH							
Southern		TREE					RUSSIAN THISTLE					
					GRASS							
						RAGWEED-SAGE						
San Francisco Bay			TREE			RAGWEED-SAGE						
						GRASS						
				DOCK-PLANTAIN								
COLORADO				TREE					SAGE			
Denver						RUSSIAN THISTLE-KOCHIA						
					GRASS		RAGWEED					
CONNECTICUT				TREE								
					GRASS							
							RAGWEED					
DELAWARE				TREE								
					GRASS							
							RAGWEED					
DIST. OF COLUMBIA				TREE								
Washington					GRASS							
							RAGWEED					
FLORIDA			TREE									
Miami				GRASS					GRASS			
						RAGWEED						
		TREE										
Tampa			GRASS									
								RAGWEED				
GEORGIA			TREE									
Atlanta						GRASS						
							RAGWEED					

Pollen calendar. From J. M. Sheldon, R. G. Lovell, K. P. Matthews, *A Manual of Clinical Allergy*, 2nd ed., 1967, W. B. Saunders, pp. 342–343. Used by permission.

Pollen calendar — pollinating seasons by state

State	Jan.	Feb.	March	April	May	June	July	Aug.	Sept.	Oct.	Nov.	Dec.
IDAHO (Southern)				TREE →				SAGE				
							RUSS THIS.-SALTBUSH					
					GRASS			RAGWEED				
ILLINOIS (Chicago)				TREE				RAGWEED				
					GRASS							
INDIANA (Indianapolis)				TREE				RAGWEED				
					GRASS							
IOWA (Ames)				TREE				RAGWEED				
					GRASS							
KANSAS (Wichita)			TREE				RUSS THIS. AMAR.					
					GRASS			RAGWEED				
KENTUCKY (Louisville)				TREE				RAGWEED				
					GRASS							
LOUISIANA (New Orleans)		TREE					GRASS					
							RAGWEED					
MAINE				TREE				RAGWEED				
					GRASS							
MARYLAND (Baltimore)				TREE				RAGWEED				
					GRASS							
MASSACHUSETTS (Boston)				TREE				RAGWEED				
					GRASS							
MICHIGAN (Detroit)				TREE				RAGWEED				
					GRASS							
MINNESOTA (Minneapolis)				TREE			CHENOPOD-AMARANTH					
					GRASS			RAGWEED				
MISSISSIPPI (Vicksburg)		TREE					GRASS					
							RAGWEED					
MISSOURI (St. Louis / Kansas City)				TREE		CHENO.-AMAR.						
					GRASS			RAGWEED				
MONTANA (Miles City)				TREE		RAGWEED-SAGE						
					GRASS							
							RUSS. THISTLE					
NEBRASKA (Omaha)				TREE		RUSS. THIST.						
					GRASS		HEMP					
							RAGWEED					
NEVADA (Reno)				TREE			RAGW.					
					GRASS		SAGE					
					RUSS.THIS -SALT BUSH							
NEW HAMPSHIRE				TREE				RAGWEED				
					GRASS							
NEW JERSEY				TREE				RAGWEED				
					GRASS							
NEW MEXICO (Roswell)			TREE				RAGWEED-SAGE					
					GRASS							
							AMARANTH-SALT BUSH					
NEW YORK (New York City)				TREE				RAGWEED				
					GRASS							

Pollen calendar chart (states and regions with active months for each allergen):

State / Region	Allergen	Active Months
NORTH CAROLINA — Raleigh	TREE	Feb.–April
	GRASS	May–June
	RAGWEED	Aug.–Sept.
NORTH DAKOTA — Fargo	TREE	April–May
	RUSSIAN THISTLE	June–Sept.
	GRASS	June–July
	SAGE	Aug.–Sept.
	RAGWEED	July–Sept.
OHIO — Cleveland	TREE	April–May
	GRASS	June–July
	RAGWEED	Aug.–Sept.
OKLAHOMA — Oklahoma City	TREE	Feb.–April
	AMARANTH	July–Sept.
	GRASS	May–Sept.
	RAGWEED	Aug.–Sept.
OREGON — Portland	TREE	March–April
	GRASS	June–July
	DOCK-PLANTAIN	June–Aug.
OREGON — East of Cascade Mountains	TREE	March–April
	GRASS	June–July
	SAGE	Aug.–Sept.
	RUSS. THIS. SLT. BSH.	July–Sept.
	RAGWEED	Aug.–Sept.
PENNSYLVANIA	TREE	April–May
	GRASS	May–June
	RAGWEED	Aug.–Sept.
RHODE ISLAND	TREE	April–May
	GRASS	June–July
	RAGWEED	Aug.–Sept.
SOUTH CAROLINA — Charleston	TREE	March–April
	GRASS	May–July
	RAGWEED	Sept.
SOUTH DAKOTA	TREE	April–May
	RUSSIAN THISTLE	July–Sept.
	GRASS	May–July
	SAGE	Aug.–Sept.
	RAGWEED	July–Aug.
TENNESSEE — Nashville	TREE	March–April
	SAGE	Sept.
	GRASS	May–Aug.
	ELM	Sept.
	RAGWEED	Aug.–Sept.
TEXAS — Dallas	TREE	Jan.–April
	ELM	Sept.
	GRASS	May–Sept.
	RAGWEED	Aug.–Oct.
	T	Dec.
TEXAS — Brownsville	GRASS	Jan.–Dec.
	AMARANTH	June–Sept.
	HACKBERRY	Feb.–April
	RAGWEED	June–Sept.
UTAH — Salt Lake City	TREE	April–May
	RUSS. THISTLE	July–Sept.
	GRASS	May–July
	SAGE	Aug.–Sept.
	RAGWEED	Aug.
VERMONT	TREE	April–May
	GRASS	June–July
	RAGWEED	Aug.–Sept.
VIRGINIA — Richmond	TREE	April–May
	GRASS	May–July
	RAGWEED	Aug.–Sept.
WASHINGTON — Seattle	TREE	March–April
	GRASS	May–Sept.
	DOCK-PLANTAIN	May–Sept.
WASHINGTON — Eastern	TREE	April–May
	SAGE	Aug.–Sept.
	GRASS	May–July
	RUSS. T. SALT BUSH	July–Sept.
	RAGWEED	Aug.
WEST VIRGINIA	TREE	April–May
	GRASS	May–July
	RAGWEED	Aug.–Sept.
WISCONSIN — Madison	TREE	April–May
	GRASS	June–July
	RAGWEED	Aug.–Sept.
WYOMING	TREE	April–May
	GRASS	June–July
	SAGE	Aug.–Sept.
	RUSSIAN THISTLE	July–Aug.
	RAGWEED	July–Aug.

Appendix E · Allergy and the Home

E1: How to Make Your Home More Allergy-Free

Hyperactivity, learning problems, and fatigue, as well as typical respiratory and cutaneous allergies can be caused by various items within your home. In a few hours or days, symptoms sometimes can be entirely relieved after making a few changes. All patients are not sensitive to all items mentioned below. What helps one patient, may not help another. If something in your home is causing symptoms, you may feel best when you are away from home, camping, or visiting. Notice if you are always worse in a certain room. The cause of your problems may reside there.

The key to an allergy-free home is to use wood, metal, glass, cotton, ceramics, and formica wherever possible. Avoid all synthetics with odors, especially plastics, polyethylene, and polyurethane. Avoid all gas appliances, oil or gas heating. Eliminate dust and do not have pets. For more information on allergy in the home see Golos 1975, Golos and Golbitz 1978, Dickey 1976a, and Maclennan 1977.

BEDROOM

More hours per day are spent in this room than in any other.

Bedding. For sheets, pillowcases, mattress pads, or blankets use only 100 percent cotton, free of chemical finishes and odor retardants. A drop of water should immediately soak into an untreated fabric. Bedspreads should be smooth, 100 percent cotton. Do not use any polyester or permanent press materials. Don't use electric blankets (plastic wiring causes odor).

Pillow. Use soft, untreated, 100 percent cotton blankets or stuff cotton diapers, cotton towels, cotton batting into 100 percent untreated, cotton pillow slips. Some patients who are not feather sensitive can use a down-filled pillow, but this can predispose one to a feather sensitivity in the future. Most new commercial down pillows are chemically treated and cannot be used. Avoid polyurethane, Dacron, Acrylon, foam rubber, kapok, or hair-filled pillows.

Mattress. Purchase a special cotton mattress cover and fill it with smooth layers of *untreated* 100 percent cotton blankets, or try a canvas army cot. Some people are sensitive to sanitized mattresses with chemical finishes and odors, mold or flame retardants, and to polyurethane or foan rubber. Old cotton mattresses in good condition might be satisfactory if enclosed in a specially constructed matress cover. For cotton mattress and pillow covers and box springs:

ECOLOGIST'S COTTON CO-OP
2986 Talisman Drive
Dallas, TX 75229

Box Springs. Use coiled type with untreated cotton cover. Avoid foam rubber.

Bed. Avoid headboards, canopy tops, bunk beds or underbed storage.

Furniture. Wood (except pine) or metal is best. Avoid ornately carved wood, Naugahyde, odorous plastic or leather, and upholstered items with synthetic filling of any type. Keep tops of dressers clear except for necessities; that is, clock, radio, lamp. Store no items with odors in dressers. Keep bookcases outside the room if possible.

Walls. Painted plaster wall, nonasbestos wall board or birch or oak paneling is best. Walls can be painted with Sherwin-Williams Soy Alkyd (Duron), Duran Alkyd paint, Du Pont's Lucite without Teflon or with casein-type paints. Add 2 ounces of baking soda to each gallon of latex-water-based paint to help reduce odors emitted from fresh paint. If preferred, walls can be covered with vinyl or nonplastic wallpaper. Prepasted wallpaper with fungicides is not advised. Use wheat starch or boiled Argo box starch with water and calcium propionate as a mold retardant. Remove old, flaking, or moldy wallpaper. Allow no fabric-covered walls, pennants, pictures, chalkboards, or dust-collecting hanging decorations. New aluminum paper is also helpful.

Windows. Use plain 100 percent cotton, silk, linen, or plain smooth shades. Avoid plastic shades, venetian blinds, ruffles, corduroy, rough textures, fiberglass or synthetic fabrics.

Floor. Best is plain wood, stone, terrazzo, smooth cement, terra cotta, or ceramic tile. Vinyl or Corlon Armstrong flooring is tolerated by some. Untreated cotton scatter rugs, nonmothproofed woolen carpets or some Sears indoor-outdoor tight weave, low nap carpets with jute backing may be tolerated. Sit directly on exact carpet to be purchased for at least half an hour, prior to purchase. Notice how you feel after such an exposure. Avoid asbestos tile or asphalt-based adhesives, plastic linoleum, hardwood finishes or waxes, synthetic odorous carpeting, shag rugs, or nylon carpets with hair (ozite), foam rubber, glue, or plastic backing.

Vacuuming. Use central vacuum cleaner with metal ducts. Water tank types are next best, but motor odors can cause symptoms. Most upright vacuums leak dust and emit motor odors.

Cleaning. Use cake Bon Ami, Borax, Arm and Hammer washing soda, Rokeach Kosher, Ivory, or pure castile soap. For heavy-duty cleaning obtain tri-sodium phosphate (Oakite) from a hardware store. Use cotton-lined "Bluette" rubber gloves for handling solution. Use ¼ cup to the two gallons water for cleaning or ½ cup per laundry load. Avoid any aerosol, pine, or phenol (Lysol) cleaning agents.

Closet. Keep only clothing worn at present time in closet. Allow no storage, mothballs, insect repellant strips, plastic garment or cleaning bags, or cedar odors. Chemical odors from freshly dry-cleaned or coin-operated cleaned clothes can cause symptoms.

LIVING ROOM

Apply same principles as used in bedroom. For children who need floor play areas, place a sheet of hard baked plastic, such as Formica, on floor in front of television. A clean 100 percent cotton blanket may be used if hard surface is not essential. Avoid odorous furniture polish.

BATHROOM

Shower Curtains. Use no plasticized fabrics. Use unfinished 100 percent cotton or terry cloth.

Shower Stall. Use tile, not plasticized substitute. Avoid synthetic glue. Or use sand and cement which is not quick drying.

Toilet Seat. Wood is best, not plastic with synthetic filling.

Cleaning. To reduce molds, clean with vinegar and water or Aqueous Zephiran (from drugstore). Allow no scented items in bathroom for cleaning or body care, hair spray, after-shaving lotion, underarm deodorant, powders, lotions, creams, shampoo, toilet, or facial tissue, etc.

KITCHEN

Stove. Corning-ware type. Use only electric, never gas, with proper ventilation and an exhaust fan.

Refrigerator Purchase electric without a self-defrost and with a minimum of plastic-coated wiring. Use baking soda to diminish odors inside refrigerator. Wipe rubber parts with vinegar to retard mold growth. Use no plastic storage containers or food bags of soft polyethylene. Store all left-over foods in glass, steel, or ceramic containers (Kailin and Brooks 1963).

Floors. Armstrong inlaid linoleum. Use no asphalt adhesive.

Table Tops. Formica or old bakelite, stainless steel, or wood.

Pots and Pans. Use stainless steel, ceramic, Pyrex, or cast-iron cooking utensils. Use no nonstick items, aluminum, plastic, or Tupperware.

Ironing Pads and Pad Covers. Must be untreated 100% cotton.

Cleaning. Allow no kitchen aerosols, floor wax, or odiferous cleaning agents.

Heating. Use electric hot-water heat with electric, not gas or oil firing, unless the heating unit and boiler are outside the home, in a separate building. Another possibility is the use of low temperature electric baseboard heat, providing the units are designed for easy vacuuming. Special international electric baseboard unpainted stainless steel heating units can be specially purchased, free of plastic and rubber parts from:

INTERTHERM. INC.
3800 Park Avenue
St. Louis, MO 63110

Solar heat is best, but impractical at the present time. Avoid oil or gas space heaters or forced-hot-air heating systems. To seal pre-existing offending heating outlets, cover them with double layers of heavy aluminum foil attached with freezer-paper tape.

Insulation. Use aluminum foil, not plastic sheeting, to cover insulation such as fiberglass.

Filters. There are several types which effectively eliminate more than 95 percent pollen, mold spores, pet hair, and dust. All have some disadvantages, however, because they can emit odors which cause symptoms in some patients. One recommended brand is supplied by:

AIR CONDITIONING ENGINEERS
Mr. H. Reed Miner
P.O. Box 616
Decatur, IL 62525

He can supply various types of charcoal and Purafil filters to help remove noxious odors, as well as dust, pollens, and molds from room air. Avoid electrostatic types unless the odor of ozone is tolerated without symptoms. Avoid high-efficiency, particulate-arresting (HEPA) filters which are ozone-free, if they emit strong chemical odors during use. These machines are costly initially, as well as for maintenance replacements. If you decide to purchase an electrostatic or HEPA unit, first sit near a functioning new unit for at least thirty minutes. Does such an exposure make you ill?

Washer and Dryer. Use only electric appliances, vented directly from basement to outside. Use Borax, baking soda, Miracle White, Ivory, or Fels Naptha soap, or Rokeach Kosher soap for cleaning. Avoid antistatic perfumed items in dryer. Avoid anticling or fabric-softener sprays. Check for bleach and laundry-item sensitivities as suggested in section E4.

E2: **Prevention and Treatment of Mold**

TO PREVENT A MOLD ALLERGY

· Purchase a dry home situated in an elevated land area. Avoid homes which need sump pumps or have basements with water-level marks on the walls indicating previous flooding.

· Avoid steaming bathroom walls from frequent hot showers. Dry damp areas after showers.

· Avoid excessive use of vaporizers in bedroom.

· Cross-ventilate and heat basement or cellar. Seal basement wall cracks with silicone· rubber seal. (Odor of seal may cause symptoms in some patients.)

· Avoid large numbers of house plants, terrariums, and home greenhouse units.

· Urge home builders to put sheets of heavy, black polyethylene under basement foundation and outside foundation wall to prevent leakage and mold problems.

· Don't rake wet leaves.

· Never leave damp clothes in washing machine or closet.

HOW TO DIMINISH MOLD CONTAMINATION IN YOUR HOME

· Remove all obviously moldy items: carpets, luggage, shoes, wallpaper, books, plants.

· Wash items or parts which appear moldy but cannot be discarded, that is, humidifiers, air-conditioners, rubber refrigerator gaskets, room vaporizers, bathroom and shower tiles, window sills, and so on. For cleaning, to protect against bacteria, molds, or fungi, use Aqueous Zephiran (from the drugstore) in a 17 percent concentration. (Dilute as directed, 1 ounce concentrate per gallon, or 1 tablespoon concentrate in 27 tablespoons water.) Be careful that it does not damage lightly varnished or finished furniture. Captan solutions: use 4 ounces powder per gallon water (from the nursery or garden-supply store). Vinegar and water may also be used, especially to reduce black mildew on refrigerator doors. One can also use quatrammonium sulphate solution or the type used in swimming pools to control algae. Borax is a good mold retardant.

· Install a dehumidifier in basement or moldy area.

E3: **Sources of Indoor Chemical Contamination**

If your child or family appears to be sensitive or made ill from odors or foods, eliminate as many of the following as possible:

Fuels. Use electric heat and cooking. Avoid hydrocarbons, that is, kerosene, coal, oil, gas, wood. These should not be in house or garage if attached. Gas appliances must be removed. It won't help if only disconnected. If heating is electric, remove motor-driven fans. These utilize oil. Use cool electric heat in form of radiator or heat pump installation with two-stage baseboard controls. Be sure there are no plastics in heating ducts. Be sure filters are not oiled. Electronic filters dry dust and can give out dangerous gases; use activated carbon filters.

Fresh Paint and Varnish and Wood Stain. Paint must be nonodorous; use Du Pont Lucite without Teflon or use Alkyd paint. Add 2 ounces baking soda per gallon.

Cements and Other Adhesives such as the following. Fingernail polish and remover, shoe polish, paint remover, hinge looseners, adhesives used in model airplanes and other toys, and floor adhesives containing tars.

Cleaning and Lighter Fluids. Be absent for several days if rugs are cleaned. Clothes should be aired in the sun after being sent to dry cleaners. No lighter fluids in the house.

Newsprint. Newspapers and magazines should be opened and read by someone else first.

Alcohol. No rubbing alcohol. No shellac or brush-cleaning preparations. No flavoring extracts such as vanilla that have alcohol in them.

Refrigerants and Spray Containers. Slow escape of gas from air conditioners or refrigerators or freezers can cause trouble. Same type gas is commonly used propellent in spray containers of insecticides, perfumes, hair sprays, and other cosmetics.

Insecticides. DDT and related compounds are usually dispensed in kerosene or other solvents. Avoid lindane, methoxychlor, DDT, chlordane, malathione, or thiocyanates. Rugs are often moth proofed with fluids containing DDT while in storage. Rug shampoo can contain DDT. Exterminators use dieldrin, chlordane, pentachlorphenal. Blankets are often moth proofed similarly. Moth balls, cakes, crystals containing naphthalene para-dichlorabenzene can cause symptoms.

Information in this section is drawn from Dr. William Rea's summary of material in *Human Ecology and the Human Environment* (Springfield, Ill.: Charles C Thomas) by Dr. Theron G. Randolph. It is used here with the kind permission of both authors.

Sponge Rubber. Odors can come from sponge rubber pillows, mattresses, upholstery, rug pads, seat cushions, typewriter pads, rubber backing of rugs, and various noise-reducing installations. Watch for restlessness, insomnia, night sweat, etc.

Plastics. The more flexible and odorous a plastic, the more frequently it contributes to indoor chemical air pollution. Hard plastics like Formica, Bakelite, cellulose acetate are rarely incriminated. Vinyl and radiant floor heating fumes should be avoided. Plastic pillows, combs, powder cases, shoes can give symptoms. Avoid plastic or fiberglass air conditioning ducts. Remove bags from clothing after dry cleaning.

Mechanical Devices. Evaporating oil from any motor. Air filters of glass wool or fiberglass usually have oiled filters, but one can get them without. Fans and motors in hot water units. Small kitchens may have too many motors. Cars in garages or near elevator shafts can volatilize gases.

Miscellaneous. Toxic fumes and odors can come from detergents, naptha-containing soaps, ammonia, Clorox, cleansing powders containing bleaches, some silver and brass polishing materials. Storage of bleach-containing cleansers. Odors of fabric softeners used in laundry dryers. Highly scented soaps, toilet deodorants, disinfectants—especially pine and scented air improvers. Phenol and other chemicals are sometimes placed in wallpaper paste. Avoid Lysol, pine Christmas trees, pine in wood-burning fireplaces, creosote odors, odors from prolonged use of TV sets, and tobacco odors.

CHEMICAL CONTAMINATION OF FOODS AND BEVERAGES

A food additive is any chemical substance that makes its way into foods. Susceptibility to chemical additives and contaminants of the diet has long been confused with specific susceptibility to foods. One may be sensitive to the food, the additive, or both. If one eats a food at one time and has no reaction, and then eats it another time and has a reaction, he probably is sensitive to the chemical and not the food. Foods commonly contaminated by chemicals are:

Foods Often Containing Spray Residues. Apples, cherries, peaches, apricots, nectarines, pears, plums, olives, currants, persimmons, strawberries, cranberry, raspberries, blueberries, boysenberries, pineapples, rhubarb, grapes, oranges, grapefruit, lemons, brussels sprouts, broccoli, cauliflower, cabbage, head lettuce, tomatoes, celery, asparagus, spinach, beet greens, chard, mustard greens, endive, escarole, leaf lettuce, romaine lettuce, Chinese cabbage, and artichokes. Most commonly used sprays permeate the food to which they are applied. They are *not* removed by washing, peeling, soaking in water or vinegar, or by cooking. Root vegetables are apt to be free of spray residues unless contaminated in transit or in the market. Lamb, beef, pork, fowl may be contaminated by the animals having eaten sprayed forage and concentrating such oil soluble insecticides, herbicides, or their vehicles in their fats. Chicken and turkey often contain residues of stilbesterol, a synthetic hormone.

Foods Often Containing Fumigant Residues. Dates, figs, shelled nuts, raisins, prunes, and other dried fruits—wheat, corn, barley, rice, dried peas, and lentils. Foods cooked in oven after use of oven cleaners.

Foods Often Containing Bleaches. White flour (unbleached flour is usually available). Freshly stone-ground whole wheat flour is much safer.

Foods Often Treated with Sulphur. Peaches, apricots, nectarines are often dusted with sulphur. Commercially prepared fresh apples, peaches, apricots, and French fried potatoes may be treated with sulphur dioxide as an antibrowning agent. Molasses, dried fruit, melon, citrus candied peel, and fruit marmalade may be bleached with sulphur dioxide. Dried apples, dried pears, dried peaches, dried apricots, raisins, prunes, corn syrup (glucose), corn sugar (dextrose), cornstarch, corn oil usually are treated with sulphur dioxide in the process of manufacture.

Foods Artificially Colored. Creme de menthe, maraschino cherries, and other colored fruit, Jell-O and other colored gelatin desserts, mint sauce, colored ice cream, colored sherbet, colored candy, colored cake, cookie and pie frostings and fillings. Weiners, bologna, cheese, butter, oleomargarine, some hamburger, some ham. Orange, sweet potato, Irish potato. Root beer, pop, cola drinks, and certain other soft and imitation drinks usually contain coal-tar dyes.

Foods Artificially Sweetened. Any containing saccharin or Sucaryl (sodium cyclamate).

Foods Exposed to Gas. Bananas are artificially ripened by exposure to ethylene gas. Apples and pears are often stored in ethylene gas. Coffee is often roasted over an open gas flame and may absorb some of the combustion products of such a flame. Cane and beet sugars usually are clarified by being filtered through bone char. These filters are usually reactivated periodically in gas-fired kilns. Absorbed combustion products apparently are imparted to the next batch of syrup which is filtered through them. Canned potato chips.

Foods Contaminated by Containers. Carrots, parsnips, turnips, tomatoes, and mixed shredded greens dispensed in odorous plastic bags. Certain other foods may also be contaminated by having been transported, stored, or frozen in plastic containers. Cellophane-wrapped foodstuffs are usually tolerated by chemically susceptible patients. In general, plastic wrappings tend to contaminate their food contents in direct proportion to the odor emitted by the wrapping material. The longer a food remains in an odorous plastic wrapping, the more it may be contaminated. Plastic refrigerator dishes for storage of foods are commonly contaminated. Citrus fruits may be contaminated by fungicide-treated containers. Foods are frequently contaminated by the golden brown lining of metal cans. This is a phenolic resin which prevents the metal from bleaching the contents of the can, but also contaminates them chemically. Only such foods as the manufacturer desires to bleach, such as asparagus, grapefruit, pineapple, artichoke, and some citrus juices, are apt to be packed in unlined cans.

Foods Often Waxed with Paraffins. Rutabagas, parsnips, turnips, peppers, cucumbers, eggplant, green peppers are waxed and lightly polished. Apples, oranges, grapefruit, tangerines, lemons are waxed and/or polished.

Foods Often Containing Desiccating Agents. Truscuit, prepared coconut—often contains added glycols.

FOODS THAT ARE LESS CHEMICALLY CONTAMINATED

Fish and Meat. Fresh or frozen seafood (lobster, crayfish, shrimp, crab, etc.). Fresh ocean, not lake, fish or fish which has been frozen in large pieces (in contrast to pound packages) are not usually contaminated. Lean meat from which the fat has been stripped prior to cooking is preferable to cooking meat with its adherent fat.

Vegetables. Fresh potatoes if undyed and home-peeled, turnips, rutabagas, eggplant, parsnips (if not waxed), squash, pumpkins, beets (tops are usually sprayed), salsify, celery root, parsley root, okra, green peas, green beans (if fresh frozen or canned in glass).

Nuts. Nuts in shell only (Brazil nuts, coconuts, walnuts, hickory nuts, pecans, filberts, hazelnuts).

Sweetening Agents. Honey, sorghum, pure maple sugar or syrup.

Fats and Oils. Olive, cottonseed, peanut, soy, coconut, sunflower, sesame, safflower—preferably cold-pressed rather than extracted by the usual solvent process, using buckwheat. Importations such as chocolate, arrowroot, tapioca, carob, and sassafras tea usually have been fumigated in shiphold. Any food may have been contaminated in transit or in markets by sprayed surroundings in contaminated bulk cartons, plastic bags, or DDT-treated burlap bags.

Most grocery-store foods are presently contaminated.

Foods from approved local sources should be secured for canning in glass or aluminum foil during the season of availability.

Membership in state or local Natural Food Associate groups or Organic Gardening Clubs is helpful in finding sources of supply.

E4: **Simple Tests for Chemical Sensitivities**

Do the following tests only if you or a family member are normally exposed to the listed items at home, school, or work. Select a time when symptoms are minimal. Never do the test on yourself. Someone must time the test and observe for possible reactions. Do test in a room which can be avoided for several hours if a reaction occurs. Discuss the test with your physician first. Test only if he approves.

Schedule the test so that it is midway between meals, at 10:00 A.M. or 3:00 P.M. Do no more than one test per day. Observe the patient for any change in activity, behavior, or the onset of symptoms—that is, flushing, pallor, stuffiness, headache, muscle ache, dizziness, and so on. Check pulse before test. If any test produces symptoms, immediately stop exposure. Breathe fresh air or oxygen. Take 1 to 2 tablespoons of baking soda in 2 glasses of water. If no reaction is noticed after the specified time of exposure, stop the test. Continue to watch the patient for an additional half hour for delayed reactions. Take pulse for one full minute every 1 to 10 minutes during entire test. Pulse increase of 12 to 20 may indicate a sensitivity to the item tested (Coca 1977).

Food Coloring

> Do not test for dyes without a physician's supervision. Severe reactions have been noted in some adults. Do not test for dyes unless all colored foods, beverages, and medicine are normally taken without obvious symptoms. Place one drop of red, grocery store food coloring under the tongue. Hold it for one minute. Then swallow. Test other colors (yellow, blue), one each day. Observe for twenty minutes. If the above is negative, give one tablespoon of colored Jell-O or artificially colored beverage each day for about five days. Observe twenty minutes after ingestion. See appendix B10 for other ways to test (Green 1974).

Shellac, turpentine, creosol, kerosene, gasoline, acetone (nail polish remover), perfume (test each one used separately), underarm deodorant, hair, body, bathroom or kitchen aerosol, perfume, Lysol, floor wax, furniture or shoe polish, camphor, pesticide, herbicide, insecticide, liquid paint, or glue

> Test each item individually.
> Place a few drops or small spray on a blotter.
> Expose patient for twenty minutes at two feet.

Clorox, ammonia, scouring powder

> Test one at a time.
> Place one tablespoon in one cup water.
> Expose patient for twenty minutes at four feet.

Foam rubber, polyurethane, soft plastic or plastic polyethylene food or garment bags, freshly cleaned or new polyester clothing:
> Test each item individually.
> Expose patient for approximately twenty minutes at two feet.

Gas fumes
> Sit two to three feet from a stove which has lighted gas burners and lighted oven for twenty to thirty minutes.
> Have doors to room closed.

Tobacco
> Sit in tobacco smoke-filled room without eating or drinking for twenty minutes.

Newsprint or chemically treated paper (mimeograph, copy machine)
> Keep freshly printed paper six inches from face for approximately twenty minutes.

Soap, detergent, or fabric softener
> Soak washcloth in usual concentration for each item. Squeeze out excess fluid.
> Keep item six inches from face for twenty minutes.
> Test each item separately.

Exhaust fumes
> Stand near busy bus stop for fifteen to twenty minutes.

Electric blanket or heating pad fumes:
> Place either on chest for twenty minutes.
> As plastic-coated wires heat, odors are emitted

Motor oils
> Stand near small motor for ten minutes.

Mothballs or crystals
> Expose patient at six feet for twenty minutes.

Carpet, linoleum, tile, upholstered furniture, mattresses or bed sheets
> Sit directly upon item for twenty to thirty minutes. Does portion of body in contact with item tingle or feel different?

Tap Water Problems

Tap water is contaminated with many substances which potentially can cause illness (Rapp 1972b, Morgan 1977).
Try various types of glass bottled spring water.
Try inspected well water, but this may contain crop or garden chemicals.
Try distilled water, but this cannot be used for prolonged periods because it lacks minerals.

Try faucet attachment or separate water line to provide filtered water. Contact:

Puro Filter Corporation
  1326 S. Michigan Avenue
  Chicago, IL 60605

Check at health food store.

To remove chlorine, boil water. To change chlorine to chloride in bath water, add one tablespoon sodium thiosulfate (from the pet store).

For more information on testing for chemical sensitivities see Golos 1975, Golos and Golbitz 1978, Dickey 1976a, and Ludeman and Henderson 1978.

References

Adler, Keif. 1976. *Beyond the Staff of Life.* Happy Camp, Calif.: Naturegraph. Wheatless-dairyless cookbook.

Alvarez, W. C. 1946. Puzzling "nervous storms" due to food allergy. *Gastroenterology* 7:241.

Barcol, A., and L. Rabkin. 1974. A precursor of delinquency—the hyperkinetic disorder of childhood. *Psychiatric Quarterly* 48:387.

Black, J. H. 1942. The treatment of food allergy. *Southern Medical Journal* 35:771.

Blume, Kathleen A. 1968. *Air Pollution in the Schools and Its Effect on Our Children.* Chicago: Human Ecology Research Foundation.

Breneman, J. C. 1978. *Basics of Food Allergy.* Springfield, Ill.: Charles C Thomas.

Breneman, J. C., et al. 1973. Report of the food-allergy committee of the American College of Allergists on the clinical evaluation of sublingual provocative testing method for diagnosis of food allergy. *Annals of Allergy* 31:382.

Brutten, M., Sylvia O. Richardson, and Charles Mangel. 1973. *Something Is Wrong with My Child.* New York: Harcourt Brace Jovanovich.

Buckley, Robert E. 1972. A neurophysiologic proposal for the amphetamine response in hyperkinetic children. *Psychosomatics* 13:93.

Buisseret, P. D. 1978. Common manifestations of cow's-milk allergy in children. *Lancet* 1:304.

Campbell, G. A. 1927. Further observations on asthma and eczema with special reference to treatment. *Canadian Medical Association Journal* 17:1498.

Cheraskin, E., W. M. Ringsdorf, Jr., and A. Brecher. 1974. *Psychodietetics.* New York: Stein & Day.

Clarke, T. Wood. 1950. The relation of allergy to character problems in children. *Psychiatric Quarterly* 24:21–38.

Cleave, T. L. 1975. *The Saccharin Disease.* New Canaan, Conn.: Keats.

Coca, Arthur F. 1977. *The Pulse Test.* New York: Arco.

Conners, C. K., C. H. Goyette, D. A. Southwick, J. M. Lees, and P. A. Andrulonis. 1976. Food additives and hyperkinesis: a controlled double-blind experiment. *Pediatrics* 58:154.

Conrad, Marion L. 1960. *Allergy Cooking.* New York: Pyramid.

Cook, P. S., and J. M. Woodhill. 1976. The Feingold dietary treatment of the hyperkinetic syndrome. *Medical Journal of Australia* 2:85.

Cooke, R. A. 1922. Studies in specific hypersensitiveness: IX. On the phenomenon of hyposensitization (the clinically lessened sensitiveness of allergy). *Journal of Immunology* 7:219.

Cott, Allan. 1977. *The Orthomolecular Approach to Learning Disabilities.* San Rafael, Cal.: Academic Therapy.

Cottrell, Edyth. 1974. *Oats, Peas, Beans, Barley.* Santa Barbara, Cal.: Woodridge Press.

Crawford, L. V., Chairman. 1976. A double-blind study of subcutaneous food testing sponsored by the Food Committee of the American Academy of Allergy. *Journal of Allergy and Clinical Immunology* 57:236.

Crook, William G. 1973. *Can Your Child Read? Is He Hyperactive?* Jackson, Tenn.: Professional.

Crook, William G. 1977. *Tracking Down Hidden Food Allergy.* Jackson, Tenn.: Professional.

Crook, William G. 1978. *Are You Allergic?* Jackson, Tenn.: Professional. Updated version of *Your Allergic Child.*

Crook, William G., W. E. Harrison, S. E. Crawford, and B. S. Emerson. 1961. Systemic manifestations due to allergy. *Pediatrics* 27:790.

Davison, H. 1949. Cerebral allergy. *Southern Medical Journal* 42:712.

Davison, H. 1952. Allergy of the nervous system. *Quarterly Review of Allergy and Applied Immunology* 6:157.

Deamer, W. C. 1971. Pediatric allergy: some impressions gained over a thirty-seven-year period. *Pediatrics* 48:930.

Deamer, William, and Oscar Frick. 1972. The allergic-tension-fatigue syndrome. *Pediatrics* 6:5.

Dickey, L. D. 1971a. Ecological illness. *Rocky Mountain Medical Journal* 68:23.

Dickey, L. D. 1971b. Sublingual antigens. *Journal of the American Medical Association* 217:214.

Dickey, L. D. 1976a. *Clinical Ecology.* Springfield, Ill.: Charles C Thomas.

Dickey, L. D. 1976b. Sublingual antigen testing and therapy for inhalants, foods, and petrochemicals. In *Clinical Ecology,* ed. L. D. Dickey, p. 544. Springfield, Ill.: Charles C Thomas.

Dohan, F. C., and J. C. Grasberger. 1973. Relapsed schizophrenics: earlier discharge from the hospital after cereal-free, milk-free diet. *American*

Journal of Psychiatry 130:6,685.

Duffy, William. 1975. *Sugar Blues*. New York: Warner.

Dworkin, Stan, and Floss Dworkin. 1974. *Natural Snacks 'n' Sweets*. Emmaus, Pa.: Rodale.

Emerling C. G., and E. O. Jonckers. 1969. *The Allergy Cookbook*. New York: Barnes and Noble.

Feingold, Ben F. 1975. *Why Your Child Is Hyperactive*. New York: Random.

Finn, R., and H. N. Cohen. 1978. Food allergy: fact or fiction? *Lancet* 1:426.

Frazier, Claude A. 1974. *Coping with Food Allergy*. New York: Quadrangle.

Fredericks, Carlton. 1976. *Psycho-nutrition*. New York: Grosset & Dunlap.

Gerrard, John W. 1973. *Understanding Allergies*. Springfield, Ill.: Charles C Thomas.

Gerras, Charles, ed. 1972. *Natural Cooking: The Prevention Way*. Emmaus, Pa.: Rodale.

Goldbeck, David, and Nikki Goldbeck. 1976. *Supermarket Handbook*. New York: New American Library.

Golos, Natalie. 1975. *Management of Complex Allergies*. Norwalk, Conn.: New England Foundation of Allergic Diseases. Large special recipe and cooking section.

Golos, Natalie, and Frances Golbitz. 1978. *Coping with Your Allergies*. New York: Simon & Schuster.

Green, Martin. 1974. Sublingual provocation testing for foods and F, D, and C dyes. *Annals of Allergy* 33:274.

Greer, Rita. 1977. *The First Clinical Ecology Cookbook*. South Sea, Hants, England: Errand Press.

Hall, Ross Hume. 1974. *Food for Nought*. New York: Vintage.

Harley, J. P. 1976. Diet and hyperactivity: any connection? *Nutrition Reviews* 34:151.

Harley, J. P., R. S. Ray, L. Tomasi, P. L. Eichman, C. G. Matthews, R. Chun, C. Cleeland, and E. Traisman. 1978. Hyperkinesis and food additives: testing the Feingold hypothesis. *Pediatrics* 61:818–827.

Hawley, Clyde, and Robert E. Buckley. 1974a. Hyperkinesis and sensitivity to the aniline food dyes. *The Journal of Orthomolecular Psychiatry* 5:129.

Hawley, Clyde, and Robert E. Buckley. 1974b. Food dyes and hyperkinetic children. *Academic Therapy* 10:27.

Hippchen, Leonard J. 1976. Biochemical approaches to offender rehabilitation. *Offender Rehabilitation* 1:115.

Hippchen, Leonard J. 1978. *The Ecologic-Biochemical Approaches to*

Treatment of Delinquents and Criminals. New York: Van Nostrand Reinhold.

Hoffer, A. 1974. Hyperactivity, allergy, and megavitamins. *Canadian Medical Association Journal* 111:905.

Hoffer, A., and H. Osmond. 1963. Malvaria, a new psychiatric disease. *Acta Psychiatrica Scandinavica* 39:335.

Hoobler, B. R. 1916. Some early symptoms suggesting protein sensitization in infancy. *American Journal of Diseases of Children* 12:129.

Human Ecology Study Group. 1977. *Very Basically Yours Cook Book.* Rev. ed. Fort Collins, Col.: Dickey.

Hunter, Beatrice Trum. 1972a. *Consumer Beware (Your Food and What's Been Done to It).* Des Plaines, Ill.: Bantam.

Hunter, Beatrice Trum. 1972b. *The Fact Book on Food Additives and Your Health.* New Canaan, Conn.: Keats.

Johnstone, D. 1957. Study of the role of antigen dosage in the treatment of pollenosis and pollen asthma. *American Journal of Diseases of Children* 94:1.

Kailin, Eloise W., and Clifton R. Brooks. 1963. Systemic toxic reactions to soft plastic food containers: a double-blind study. *Medical Annals of District of Columbia* 32:1.

Keston, Beatrice, Irene Waters, and J. Gardner Hopkins. 1935. Oral desensitization to common foods. *Journal of Allergy* 6:431.

Kittler, F. G., and D. G. Baldwin. 1970. The role of allergic factors in the child with minimal brain dysfunction. *Annals of Allergy* 28:203.

Lee, Carlton H., Russell I. Williams, and Edward Binkley. 1969. Provocative testing and treatment for foods. *Archives of Otolaryngology* 90:113.

Leonard, Jon N., J. L. Hofer, and N. Pritikin. 1974. *Live Longer Now . . . The First 100 Years of Your Life.* New York: Grosset & Dunlap.

Levy, Harold B. 1973. *Square Pegs-Round Holes.* Boston: Little, Brown.

Lockey, S. D. 1971. Reactions to hidden agents in foods, beverages, and drugs. *Annals of Allergy* 29:461.

Lockey, S. D. 1977. Hypersensitivity to tartrazine (F, D, and C yellow #5) and other dyes and additives present in foods and pharmaceutical products. *Annals of Allergy* 38:206.

Ludeman, Kay, and Louis Henderson. 1978. *Resource Handbook on Allergies.* Dallas, Tex.: Human Ecology Research Association.

Mackarness, Richard. 1976. *Eating Dangerously.* New York: Harcourt Brace Jovanovich.

Maclennan, John. 1977. *Common Sense for the Sensitive.* Hamilton, Ontario: Human Ecology Foundation of Canada.

Mandell, Marshall. 1977. Cerebral reactions in allergic patients. In *A*

Physician's Handbook on Orthomolecular Medicine, ed. R. J. Williams and D. K. Kalita. Elmsford, N.Y.: Pergamon.

Marks, M. B. 1977. *Physical Signs of Allergy of the Respiratory Tract in Children*. Kalamazoo, Mich.: Upjohn.

Mayron, L. W., J. Ott, R. Nations, and E. L. Mayron. 1974. Light, radiation, and academic behavior. *Academic Therapy* 10:33.

Mednick, S. 1966. A longitudinal study of children with a high risk for schizophrenia. *Mental Hygiene* 50:4.

Mendelson, W., N. Johnson, and M. A. Stewart. 1971. Hyperactive children as teen-agers: a follow-up study. *Journal of Nervous and Mental Disease* 153:273.

Menkes, M. M., J. S. Rowe, and J. H. Menkes. 1967. A twenty-five-year follow-up study on the hyperkinetic child with minimal brain dysfunction. *Pediatrics* 39:393.

Miller, Joseph B. 1972. Food Allergy: *Provocative Testing and Injection Therapy*. Springfield, Ill.: Charles C Thomas.

Miller, Joseph B. 1977. A double-blind study of food extract injection therapy: a preliminary report. *Annals of Allergy* 38:185–191.

Millman, M. M., M. B. Campbell, K. Wright, and A. Johnston. 1976. Allergy and learning disability in children. *Annals of Allergy* 36:149.

Morgan, Joseph. 1977. The water problem. In *Clinical Ecology*, ed. L. D. Dickey, pp. 306–309. Springfield, Ill.: Charles C Thomas.

Morris, D. L. 1969. Use of sublingual antigen in diagnosis and treatment of food allergy. *Annals of Allergy* 27:289.

Morrison, J. R., and M. A. Stewart. 1971. A family study of the hyperactive syndrome. *Biological Psychiatry* 3:3,189.

Moyer, K. E. 1975. The physiology of violence, allergy, and aggression. *Psychology Today* 9:76.

Moyer, K. E. 1976. *The Psychobiology of Aggression*. New York: Harper.

Newbold, H. L. 1975. *Meganutrients for Your Nerves*. New York: Wyden.

Nichols, Joe D. 1974. *Please, Doctor, Do Something*. Atlanta, Tex.: Natural Food Associates.

Nizami, Riaz M., Peter K. Lewin, and M. Toyer Baboo. 1977. Oral cromolyn therapy in patients with food allergy: a preliminary report. *Annals of Allergy* 39:102.

O'Banion, D., B. Armstrong, and R. H. Cummings. 1978. Disruptive behavior: a dietary approach. *Journal of Autism and Childhood Schizophrenia* 8:325.

O'Shea, James. 1978. Sublingual immunotherapy of hyperkinetic children with food, chemical and inhalent allergens: a double-blind study. Paper presented at the Twelfth Advanced Seminar in Clinical Ecology at Key Biscayne, Florida, November 1978.

Oski, Frank. 1977. *Don't Drink Your Milk*. New York: Wyden.

Ott, John. 1976. *Health and Light*. New York: Pocket Books.

Pfeiffer, Carl. 1975. *Mental and Elemental Nutrients*. New Canaan, Conn.: Keats.

Philpott, William H. 1977. Maladaptive reactions to frequently used food and commonly met chemicals as precipitating factors in many chronic physical and chronic emotional illnesses. In *A Physician's Handbook on Orthomolecular Medicine*, ed. R. J. Williams and D. K. Kalita. Elmsford N.Y.: Pergamon.

Prevention Magazine Editors. 1972. *Natural Cooking the Prevention Way*. Emmaus, Pa.: Rodale. Milk-free, sugar-free, and many wheat-free recipes.

Randolph, Theron G. 1947. Allergy as a causative factor of fatigue, irritability, and behavior problems of children. *Journal of Pediatrics* 31:560.

Randolph, Theron G. 1950. Specific food allergens in alcoholic beverages. *Journal of Laboratory and Clinical Medicine* 36:976–977.

Randolph, Theron G. 1962. *Human Ecology and Susceptibility to the Chemical Environment*. Springfield, Ill.: Charles C Thomas.

Randolph, Theron G. 1976a. The enzymatic, acid, hypoxia, endocrine concept of allergic inflammation. In *Clinical Ecology*, ed. L. D. Dickey, pp. 577–596. Springfield, Ill.: Charles C Thomas.

Randolph, Theron G. 1976b. The role of specific alcoholic beverages. In *Clinical Ecology*, ed. L. D. Dickey, pp. 321–333. Springfield, Ill.: Charles C Thomas.

Rapaport, Howard G., and Shirley H. Flint. 1976. Is there a relationship between allergy and learning disabilities? *Journal of School Health* 46:139.

Rapp, Doris J. 1972a. *Allergies and Your Child*. New York: Holt, Rinehart & Winston.

Rapp, Doris J. 1972b. Water as a cause of angio-edema and urticaria. *Journal of the American Medical Association* 218:221–305.

Rapp, Doris J. 1974. *Questions and Answers about Allergies and Your Child*. Sterling, 2 Park Ave., New York, N.Y. 10016

Rapp, Doris J. 1978a. Double-blind confirmation and treatment of milk sensitivity. *Medical Journal of Australia* 4:571–572.

Rapp, Doris J. 1978b. Does diet affect hyperactivity? *Journal of Learning Disability* 11:56–62.

Rapp, Doris J. 1978c. Food allergy treatment for hyperkinesis. *Journal of Learning Disabilities* 11/79.

Rapp, Doris J. 1978d. Weeping eyes in wheat allergy. *Transactions of the American Society of Ophthalmology and Otolaryngology* 18: 149-151, 1978.

Rea, William J. 1976. Environmentally triggered thrombophlebitis. *Annals of Allergy* 37:101.

Rea, William J. 1977. Environmentally triggered small-vessel vasculitis. *Annals of Allergy* 38:245.

Rea, William J. 1978. Environmentally triggered cardiac disease. *Annals of Allergy* 40:243.

Rinkel, Herbert J. 1944. Food allergy: the role of food allergy in internal medicine. *Annals of Allergy* 2:115.

Rinkel, Herbert J., C. H. Lee, D. W. Brown, J. W. Willoughby, and J. M. Williams. 1964. The diagnosis of food allergy. *Archives of Otolaryngology* 79:71.

Rinkel, H., T. Randolph, and M. Zeller. 1951. *Food Allergy*. Norwalk, Conn.: New England Foundation of Allergic and Environmental Diseases.

Robins, L. M. 1966. *Deviant Children Grow Up: A Sociological and Psychiatric Study of Sociopathic Personality*. Baltimore: Williams and Wilkins.

Rosenberg, Harold, and A. N. Feldzamen. 1974. *The Doctor's Book of Vitamin Therapy*. New York: Putnam.

Roth, June. 1977. *Cooking for Your Hyperactive Child*. Chicago, Ill.: Contemporary.

Roth, June. 1978. *The Food Depression Connection*. Chicago, Ill.: Contemporary.

Rowe, A. H. 1950. Allergic toxemia and fatigue. *Annals of Allergy* 8:72.

Rowe, A. H. 1959. Allergic toxemia and fatigue. *Annals of Allergy*. 17:9.

Rowe, Albert, and Albert Rowe, Jr. 1972. *Food Allergy*. Springfield, Ill.: Charles C Thomas.

Sainsbury, Isobel S. 1974. *The Milk-Free and Milk-Free, Egg-Free Cookbook*. Springfield, Ill.: Charles C Thomas.

Salzman. L. K. 1976. Allergy testing, psychological assessment, and dietary treatment of the hyperactive child syndrome. *Medical Journal of Australia* 2:248.

Sandberg, D. H., D. W. Bernstein, R. M. McIntosh, R. Carr, and J. Strauss. 1977. Severe steroid-responsive nephrosis associated with hypersensitivity. *Lancet* 8008:388–391.

Schloss, O. M. 1912. A case of allergy to common foods. *American Journal of Diseases of Children* 111:341.

Schofield, A. T. 1908. A case of egg poisoning. *Lancet* 1:716.

Schroeder, Henry A. 1973. *Trace Elements and Man*. Old Greenwich, Conn.: Devin-Adair.

Schroeder, Henry A. 1974. *The Poisons Around Us: Toxic Metals in Food, Air and Water*. Bloomington: Indiana University Press.

Shaywitz, B. A., J. R. Goldenring, and R. S. Wool. 1978. Effects of chronic administration of food colorings on activity levels and cognitive performance in normal and hyperactive developing rat pups. *Annals of Neurology* 4: 196.

Simeon, Jovan, et al. 1978. Cromolyn DSG effects in hyperkinetic and psychotic children with allergies. Paper presented at the Second International Food Allergy Symposium, at Mexico City, October 1978.

Singh, Man Mohan, and Stanley R. Kay. 1976. Wheat gluten as a pathenogenic factor in schizophrenia. *Science* 191:401.

Speer, F. 1954. Allergic tension-fatigue in children. *Annals of Allergy* 12:168.

Speer, F. 1970. *Allergy of the Nervous System*. Springfield, Ill.: Charles C Thomas.

Speer, F., and R. Dockhorn. 1973. *Allergy and Immunology in Children*. Springfield, Ill.: Charles C Thomas.

Stewart, Mark A., and Sally Olds. 1973. *Raising the Hyperactive Child* New York: Harper.

Stone, Irwin. 1974. *The Healing Factor*. New York: Grosset & Dunlap.

Swanson, J. M. 1978. Behavioral response to artificial color. Paper presented at the Second International Food Allergy Symposium, at Mexico City, October 1978.

Swanson, J. M., M. Kinsbourne, and W. Roberts. 1976. Stimulant-related state dependent learning in hyperactive children. *Pediatric Research* 10:4,304.

Taube, E. Louis. 1973. *Food Allergy and the Allergic Patient*. Springfield, Ill.: Charles C Thomas.

Trites, Ronald W., H. Tryphonas, and B. Ferguson. 1978. Treatment of hyperactivity in a child with allergies to food. In *Case Studies in Hyperactivity*, ed. Marvin J. Fine. Springfield, Ill.: Charles C Thomas (in press).

Tuft, Louis. 1973. *Allergy Management in Clinical Practice*. St. Louis, Mo.: Mosby.

von Hilsheimer, George. 1970. *How to Live with Your Special Child*. Washington, D.C.: Acropolis.

von Hilsheimer, George. 1974. *Allergy, Toxins, and the Learning Disabled Child*. San Rafael, Cal.: Academic Therapy.

Wacker, John A. 1974. *The Reduction of Crime Thru the Prevention and Treatment of Learning Disabilities*. Available through author, Box 20445, Dallas, TX 75220.

Weiss, Jules M., and Herbert S. Kaufman. 1971. A subtle organic component in some cases of mental illness. *Archives of General Psychiatry* 25:74.

Wender, Esther. 1977. Food additives and hyperkinesis. *American Journal of Diseases of Children* 131:1204.

Wender, Paul. 1973. Some speculations concerning a possible biochemical basis of minimal brain dysfunction. *Annals of The New York Academy of Science* 205:18.

Williams, I. J., D. M. Cram, M. Douglas, F. T. Tausig, and E. Webster. 1978. Relative effects of drugs and diet on hyperactive behaviors: an experimental study. *Pediatrics* 61:811–817.

Williams, Roger J., and Dwight K. Kalita. 1977. *A Physician's Handbook on Orthomolecular Medicine.* Elmsford, N.Y.: Pergamon.

Willoughby, J. W. 1974. Serial dilution titration skin tests in inhalant allergy. *Otolaryngologic Clinics of North America* 7:579.

Wood, Marion. 1972a. *Delicious and Easy Rice Flour Recipes.* Springfield, Ill.: Charles C Thomas.

Wood, Marion. 1972b. *Gourmet Food on a Wheat-Free Diet or Delicious and Easy Rice Recipes.* Springfield, Ill.: Charles C Thomas.

Wunderlich, Ray C. 1973. *Allergy, Brains and Children Coping.* St. Petersburg, Fla.: Johnny Reads.

Yaryura-Tobias, J. A., and F. A. Neziroglu. 1975. Violent behavior, brain dysrhythmia, and glucose dysfunction: a new syndrome. *Journal of Orthomolecular Psychiatry* 4:182.

Reference Index

General Index